BABY BUMP

2

ADRENALINE JUMP

Stories of Ordinary Mothers with Extraordinary Achievements

Disha Shrivastava

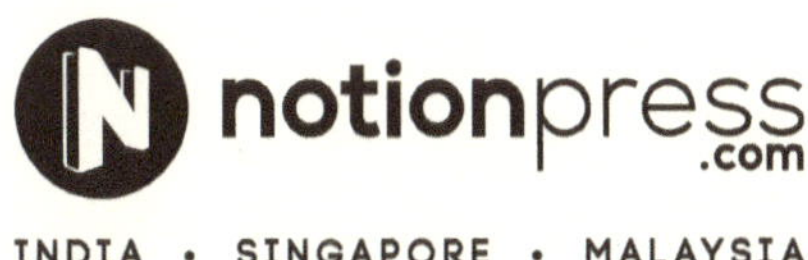

INDIA • SINGAPORE • MALAYSIA

Notion Press Media Pvt Ltd

No. 50, Chettiyar Agaram Main Road,
Vanagaram, Chennai, Tamil Nadu – 600 095

First Published by Notion Press 2021
Copyright © Disha Shrivastava 2021
All Rights Reserved.

ISBN 978-1-63806-783-2

श्री कृष्णार्पणमस्तु

Dedication

To every single mother who has somehow and somewhere lost herself in the name of motherhood, duties & responsibilities and is trying to find her spark.

To Sid, Abhi and Tango for calling me, Mamma.

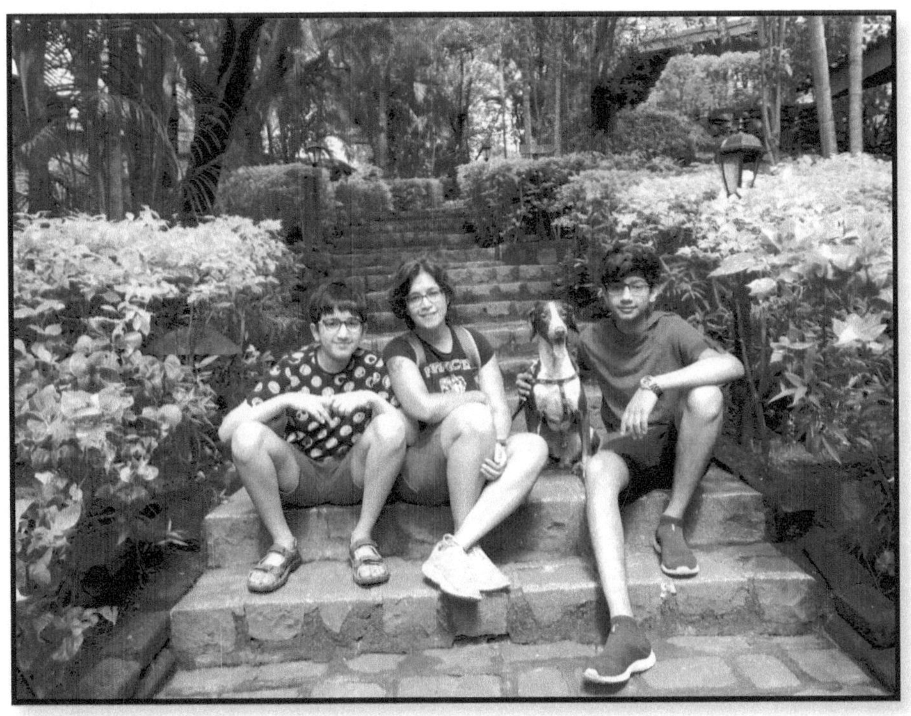

The Story Behind the Logo

(Designed by Dubai based Trimom, Chandani Desai)

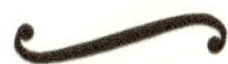

- ➤ The logo talks about the journey of a TriMom.

- ➤ The round shape is the wheel of the bicycle, denoting a cycling lap in a Triathlon.

- ➤ Inside the wheel, there is a drop-shaped womb, denoting the swim lap in a Triathlon.

- ➤ The tiny shoes inside the womb denote the running lap in a Triathlon.

- ➤ The hand holds the womb carefully, depicting a mother's gentleness yet her strength to achieve the impossible and shielding her baby.

- ➤ The umbilical cord coiling to form the number "2", depicts the forever connect and the energy between the mother and her baby.

Contents

Foreword

Disha is one person who doesn't know the meaning of impossible. When I picked her for the Passion Trail cycling expedition in Bhutan, it was due to the commitment that she demonstrated during the selection process.

But that was just the start. She is a transformed person ever since. Takes her fitness as seriously and passionately as anyone else I know and will push the envelope to achieve what would seem tough for most.

Even though I have followed her fitness journey closely, it is still something that I would love to read about again and again, as would all others who don't know about it yet!

– Rajesh Kalra
Executive Chairman at
Asianet News Media & Entertainment Pvt Ltd

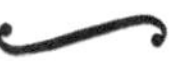

This book is going to be very inspiring to read, for both genders of athletes.

Women have proved time and again that they are very good in endurance sports.

"If I quit, everybody's going to believe women can't do this."

That was the thought that latched itself into Kathrine Switzer's head when a male official tried to push her off the course of the Boston Marathon in 1967. In spite of feeling scared and ashamed thinking she has done anything wrong, she continued running and crossed the finish line in 4h 20min.

Take for instance Frances Hayward, the first woman to run the Comrades in 1923, her entry was refused, so she was an unofficial entrant. She completed the event in 11:35 and although she was not awarded a Comrades medal, the other runners and spectators presented her with silver tea service and a rose bowl.

These women created history and we are very proud of our women athletes. They are multi-taskers and stand at par with male athletes. This book carries the stories of women, who have defied the odds and have set a path for others to follow. It's going to be very interesting to read. As a coach, I have seen that women who are consistent are very good learners. I hope this book inspires and motivates everyone who reads it. Kudos to Disha for bringing out the story and my good wishes to Disha for the success of this book.

– Satish Gujaran
Director at Network TwentyOne/Ultra Marathoner,
First Indian to finish 10 consecutive Comrades Marathon and
felicitated with Green Number. Motivational Speaker.
(Disha's running coach)

Amongst endurance sports, Triathlons have been the most challenging. This is what attracted me to doing them and eventually stepping into the coaching world.

It is never easy to excel in a single sport let alone claim to be good at all three sports. Also the investment needed to pursue this sport is high, both in terms of monetary and dedication. The determination to participate in a triathlon has to come from within, otherwise training for one becomes a chore. Many of the triathletes that I have coached take up the sport for different reasons. But there is one trait common in all, the willingness to do what's needed to reach the finish line.

Disha got in touch with me in June of 2018 with loads of enthusiasm. On her list was an Olympic Distance Triathlon, a Half Marathon in September and one more in December. She was always interested in understanding the finer points in training be it the zones or the assessment tests

Training Disha was never about pushing her to do better but more of guiding her and encouraging her to pursue her races. It was more about setting up a training plan around her busy schedule to ensure that she enjoys her training and participation in races. Time was of essence and she had to balance her kids, school, work, travel and train. Beside juggling all of the above she also managed to cycle across Italy!

Her journey to completing a Triathlon wasn't easy. The fear of Open water swimming and mass starts was intimidating. We went back to the drawing board to redefine her training, swim speed before deciding to participate in the Abu Dhabi triathlon.

While she was training for her Triathlon, she did a few Half Marathons, completing the NEB Mumbai HM, Airtel Delhi HM and the Singapore HM in 2018. She then did a few Open Water swims to get her confidence up, the HTHM and the BNP Ultra while training for her A race (the Abu Dhabi Triathlon).

On March 9, 2019 Disha finally completed her first triathlon. It brought me immense satisfaction in seeing her succeed. Hope you find inspiration when reading this book to achieve your own goals and milestones.

– Viv Menon
Disha's Triathlon Coach

I first met Disha more than a decade ago, when she was the mother for 2 toddlers confined to her house. I was working for a large software MNC in a leadership role. I was driving a CSR initiative and that's when I met her as a volunteer. She had a lot of ideas, energy, and showed unconditional love for people. She wanted to create some impact on the society at large. She was especially passionate about educating the underprivileged and empowering women.

There was a point in her life when she was not in the best of her shape; physically and mentally. She had to work very hard on herself. She gradually embraced running & cycling as part of her rigorous fitness regime. Got her physical fitness in top condition. She is a person who was willing to adventure, and charter into unexplored territories. She learnt to swim in open waters and also participated in triathlons. This feat can be achieved by very few people who are physically and mentally fit. Over the years she has been a huge pillar of strength for women in distress. She has helped several women to get out of the cocoon, push them out of their comfort zone and perform miracles.

I as her friend, mentor & coach have seen how she has transformed herself over the last decade and also helped other women go through a journey of self-discovery & change for the better.

I am glad to see that she has leveraged her multiple talents and her own personal experiences to author this book. You will be inspired to know how some of the ordinary mothers, who have done extraordinary things, otherwise would have sacrificed their personal ambition to take care of the family. They would have never known what was possible for them in their lives.

True to the meaning of her name, "Disha" will help you get direction in your life; once you read this book and put the learning into practice.

– Srikanth
B, Tech (Hons,) IIT, Kharagpur, Professional Certified Coach
(International Coaching Federation)
coachsrikanth.com
Bangalore

I first met Disha in our Bhutan cycling expedition in 2015. Her zeal, enthusiasm and never to give up attitude makes her distinguished. The way she has progressed in her fitness journey is remarkable. I am sure she'll do wonders with this book as well.

– Ankit Bhatnagar
Senior Computer Scientist, Adobe
Delhi

I met Disha during a cycling trip to Bhutan in 2015, she was a weak rider then who was struggling with riding and now She has turned up to be a triathlete with excellent endurance. Her growth as an athlete and individual is inspiring.

– Manish Mishra
Senior Auditor
PAG(AUDIT-1)U.P.
Allahabad

The cycling trip to Bhutan was a stepping stone to Disha and since then it's no looking back. She is the epitome not only for endurance training but also for organising cycle trips across the world, a pathway for others to find themselves from within

– Kavit Shah
Supply chain Consultant, Blue Yonder,
Bangalore

Words would be less to express my feelings to define "Transformed Disha". She is a fighter, has outgrown her fears to become bolder. She is a Bravo!!!

– Raj Kamal Chauhan
Managing Director
EVISU India Pvt Ltd
Gurgaon

You had always been my inspiration during our time in Bhutan. I remember I'd be struggling to get going at 5 am for our whole day cycling trips, with sleepy look on my face yet there you were there wide-awake, full of energy, smiling and vibing and all ready to start the challenge. That was beautiful and inspiring to observe.

– Abhimanyu Grover
Founder, GameB Ventures
Location: Planet Earth

Disha is a go-getter and her diligent approach impressed me. Her interest in social impact, sustainability and fitness was an interesting combination and she has managed to achieve so much in this space. She is very articulate in her communication and a great conversationalist. She briefed me about the book and I can't wait to read it.

– Debabrat (Debu) Mishra
Helping business leaders and startup founders create a lasting legacy
Mumbai

Gratitude. That's the word that comes to me for Disha. Disha is a woman who believes in herself. She has brought so much into my life, helped me in significant ways. Disha is determined to support women everywhere, and I am so grateful to have had the opportunity to support me. I have never met you, but you have touched my soul. It was hard for me to come back without your strength.

Bless You, Always.

– Megha Dhiman
System Manager – Ericsson AB
Sweden

Preface

"After all those years as a woman hearing 'not thin enough, not pretty enough, not smart enough, not this enough, not that enough,' almost overnight I woke up one morning and thought: I'm enough." – Anna Quindlen

A child gives birth to a mother, and my belief in womanhood became assertive after my kids.

The responsibility to nurture and bring up tiny humans is tenacious as well as delicate.

In this entire process of motherhood, we tend to forget ourselves. Our liking and priorities take a back seat.

Do you even remember when the last time you prepared a full meal of your choice?

Do you remember the last time you had a relaxed day?

Do you remember not being guilty because your kid didn't score well in exams?

After a horrible episode of postpartum depression, I took a conscious decision to divert my energy and tame the negative thoughts to athletics. Endurance training didn't just help make me physically tough but gave a proper direction to my mind.

In the same journey, I came across a group at Facebook, IndianWomensTriathlonClub. As I traversed through the posts, I realised that all mothers face a similar dilemma of time management, family duties, society pressures and stereotypes.

Hence the idea originated to write about Indian Tri Moms.

I wanted to tell stories of these ordinary mothers who have fought their own battle and have accomplished the extraordinary.

It takes nine months to nurture a living being and deliver. Childbirth is a phenomenal event, and this book took exactly nine months from conception to delivery.

The IndianTriMoms have shared real-life stories, some secrets, struggles, hard work and triumph.

Give this newborn lots of love.

Grateful for you for making this book a part of your reading collection.

Acknowledgements

Writing stories of personal achievements is more than an experience. It's a life-changing phenomenon to me.

Thanks, all you Indian Tri Moms, for sharing your journey and making me a secret keeper.

Thanks, Deepa, for being there in all my outbursts.

Thanks, Pradeep, for listening to me patiently and to all the blabbering.

Thanks, Srikanthan, for making me realise my strength when I had almost given all hope.

Thanks, Sid and Abhi, for a tight hug after my long writing hours. Som for arranging necessary equipment for Instalive sessions. My pet Tango for not barking during interviews.

Significant thanks to Jowana Aunty, my full-time help. I would have never written a single word without her.

Thanks, Jigna, for helping me copy editing this book.

Thanks to the small tiny virus that jolted the entire world and I was no exception. With a source of income becoming nil, writing this book and talking to other Tri moms kept me sane.

Thanks, Papa, for putting the idea of writing a book a long time back. I hope I did justice.

To the universe to make this happen despite all odds.

Bull's Eye | 01

Kirti Virmani, Gurgaon

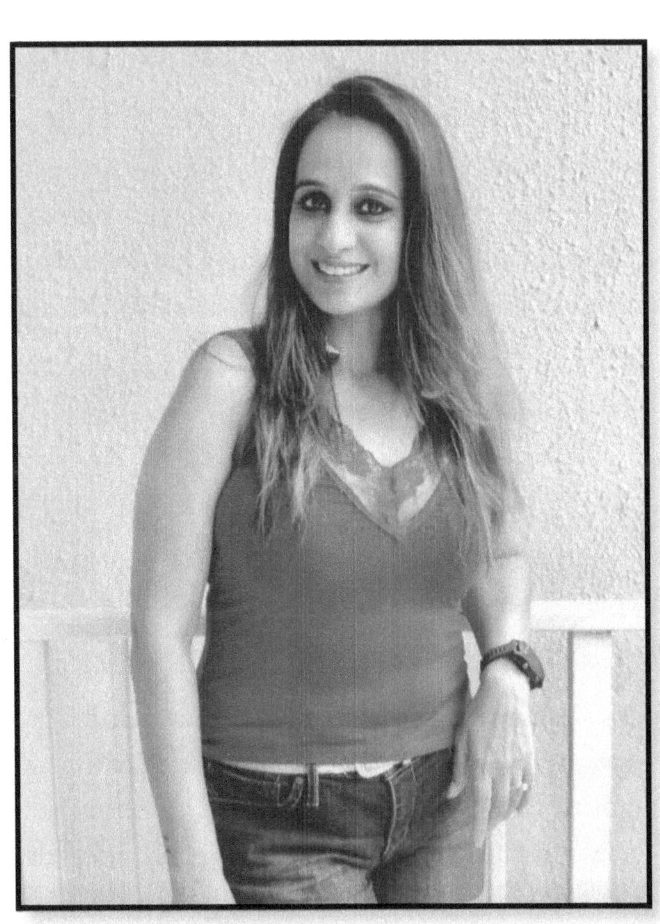

It was her decision. She made up her mind. She took the first step. And then many more. Because as you'll read in her story, Kirti Virmani doesn't shy away from a new challenge; not anymore.

Gurgaon-based, 42-year-old Virmani is a Super Randonneur (SR) title holder, winner of many cycling races, Delhi International Triathlon (DIT) (70.3, second position), a podium finisher in sprints and Olympic-distance triathlons, among others. This is her story.

Household Chores to Running Shoes

I was born in Bhiwani, Haryana. After completing my M.Sc in Mathematics, I got married in 2001. Soon after, I had my first child. Domestic responsibilities kept me away from pursuing a career and I got absorbed in household chores.

In 2007, we shifted to Gurgaon from Yamunanagar. I was keen to have another child, but I suffered from secondary infertility. I went through IVF and delivered a baby girl in 2012. It was a long gap between my two children. A decade to be precise. I had put on a lot of weight, and the IVF process left me completely drained out.

Managing two kids with a significant age difference was nothing less than a roller coaster ride. They had different demands and needs from me. My life revolved around my kids and my home. The responsibility was exhausting me. I wanted an outlet to release my stress. Moreover, I had put on a lot of weight due to my pregnancy. It was disturbing to see myself in the mirror, to say the least.

I used to take my kids for a morning stroll and there I saw young girls running in groups. I saw this every day. On the weekends, the numbers were larger. Upon inquiring about the running groups, I came to know about Pinkathon. I knew I had to join the group. And join, I did. I also started with power yoga and started regaining my energy levels.

I joined the running group for two reasons – to have a social circle of like-minded people and to build running stamina. I started loving the change and welcomed it enthusiastically. I didn't need an alarm to wake up in the morning. I was up on my own. And before my family woke up and the house buzzed with activity, I was back, fully charged up to carry out the daily chores.

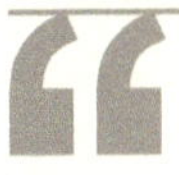

"In giving birth to our babies, we may find that we give birth to new possibilities within ourselves."

Myla and Jon Kabat-Zinn

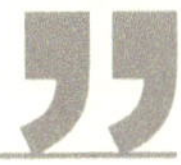

Wheelspin

In July 2015, I joined Gurgaon Road Runner, a running group. I was a newbie to running and a slow runner while the group was filled with avid runners. I felt out of place. So I switched to cycling. Cycling gave me a good kick. I felt liberated while cycling.

Within a few months, I felt stronger than before and ready for my first 50 km ride. It took around three to four hours to complete the ride, but I was on cloud nine! There was no looking back after this.

In 2016, I did my longest rides – one from Gurgaon to Jaipur, which was 200 km, and the other to Timber Trail, which was 300 km. Around the same time, a member of the running group proposed a cycle ride from Manali to Leh.

Alok, my husband, always supported me and accompanied me on all my rides. I had never done any long-distance ride without him. He too had started running and cycling for fitness but was not keen to join the Manali-Leh ride. I had a tough choice to make.

He encouraged me to go ahead with the ride, and I mustered the courage to pack my bags and embark on this epic ride. Alas! I could not complete the ride as I missed Alok, so much so that I fell sick. But this trip also gave me teammates and friends that I'm grateful for, especially Nitin Yadav, who took care of me and accompanied me to that high altitude.

"A real friend is one who walks in when the rest of the world walks out."

Walter Winchell

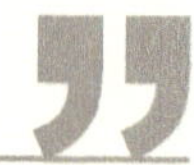

Once back from the trip, I registered for the Golden Triangle tour (Delhi-Agra-Jaipur-Delhi, 750 km in three days). It was a great learning experience for me, full of adventures. We rode in the dark, lost our way, got chased by boys, fixed punctures, and so much more.

I also completed my SR series in due course of time. Till now, I was clueless about the types of bikes available in the market as I did the SR series on my 17-kg hybrid bike. I started gathering podiums in many races and my cycle wheel was spinning in full glory.

The Tri Entry: Better Late Than Never

In the desire to add variety to my workout, I thought of learning to swim. I started with proper guided coaching classes from July 2019 and attempted my first sprint triathlon in August 2019. I grabbed a podium in this race.

Going ahead, I registered for the Olympic-distance in October. But there was one point of worry – the event was in a 16-meter pool while I had always practiced in a five-meter pool. On the day of the race, as I had thought, I panicked due to the depth of the pool. But not attempting it was not even a thought.

I composed myself and requested the organizers to allow me to settle down. Once calm, I started the swim. I completed the race beyond the cut-off time, and it was a swim DNF (Did Not Finish). I am grateful to the organizers to not stop me from finishing the race. I knew my weak point now and what had to be improved.

In February 2020, I attempted the 70.3 distance triathlon organized by Delhi International Triathlon. DIT will remain an exceptional race to me, firstly, because of the distance, and secondly, I completed this race under immense mental stress.

I was under tremendous pressure when I stepped on the start line. I started to throw up after the 11th km in the run course but was determined to finish it. Seeing my family and friends at the finish line was a great relief. I stood second in the race.

I took a significant decision and registered for Ironman 70.3, Austria in May 2020. Although the race didn't take place due to the pandemic, I was adamant about overcoming my fear of open water. I enrolled myself for open water swim sessions in Goa and was looking forward to training under proper guidance.

Neither could I attend the swimming training in Goa, nor could I attempt Ironman, but the decision to attempt the race has filled me with a lot of self-confidence. The races also helped me in strengthening my mind and getting over stress and anxiety quickly.

When God Gives You Lemons, Squeeze Them Into Tequila

I remember the days when I was immersed in household chores and responsibilities. I had no time for myself and gave every bit to my home.

During a crisis in my husband's business, we were left with mere survival capital. I pitched in and started working to contribute to the household. My husband never fails to mention that the best thing I did during those hard times was, to stay back.

After all the years of struggle and tough times, both Alok and I have stood as the strongest pillars for ourselves and our children. Alok encouraged and supported me in my passion, and I left no stone unturned to churn the best from every possibility.

I waited patiently, for I knew that the cocoon will take its own time to crack open and the butterfly will be out in the open.

Tough Times Don't Last, Tough People, Do

For all the women who are feeling stuck or are unable to muster the courage to stand for themselves, remember, no one else will do it for you. You have to take that first step and keep moving ahead, the universe will conspire to make it happen for you.

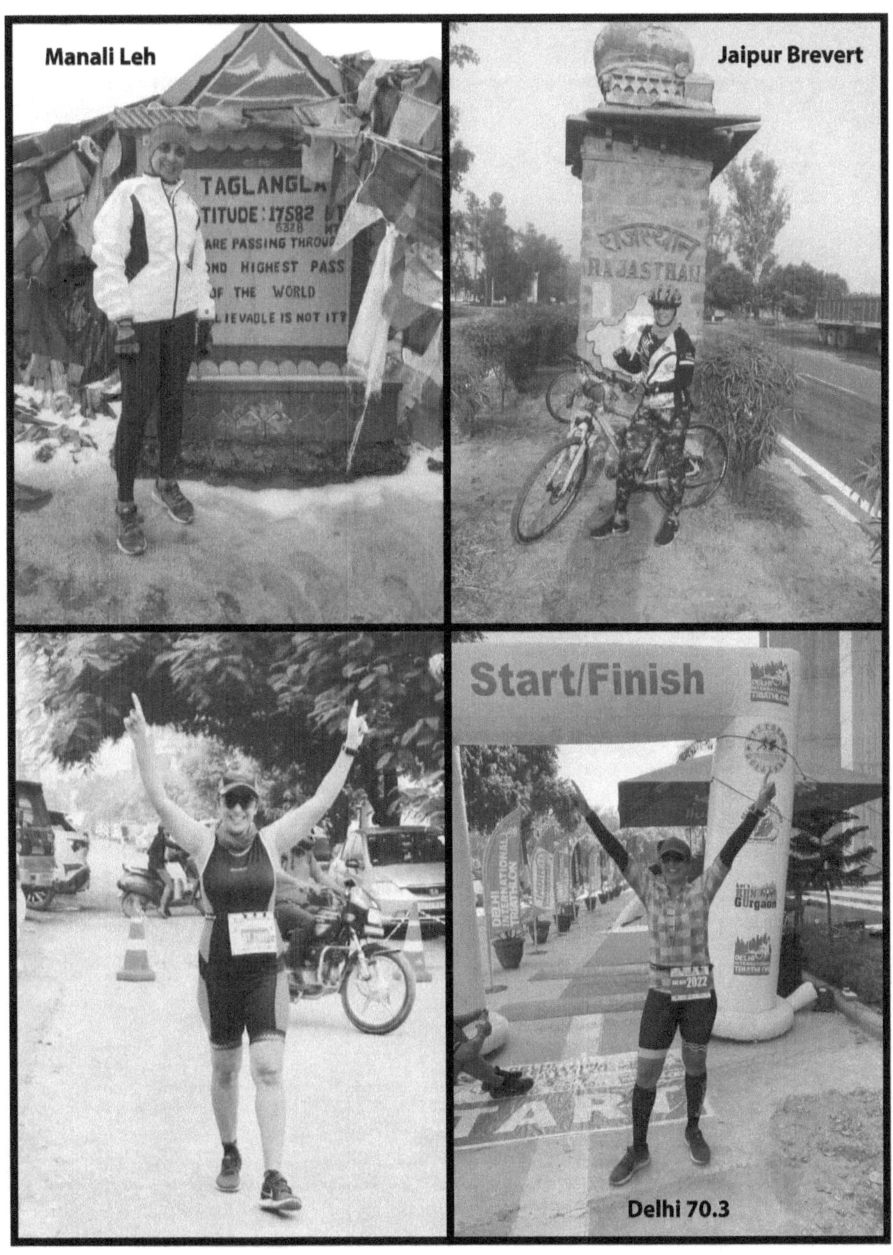
Manali Leh
TAGLANGLA
TITUDE : 17582
5328
ARE PASSING THROU
ND HIGHEST PASS
OF THE WORLD
LIEVABLE IS NOT IT?
Jaipur Brevert
RAJASTHAN
Start/Finish
Gurgaon
Delhi 70.3

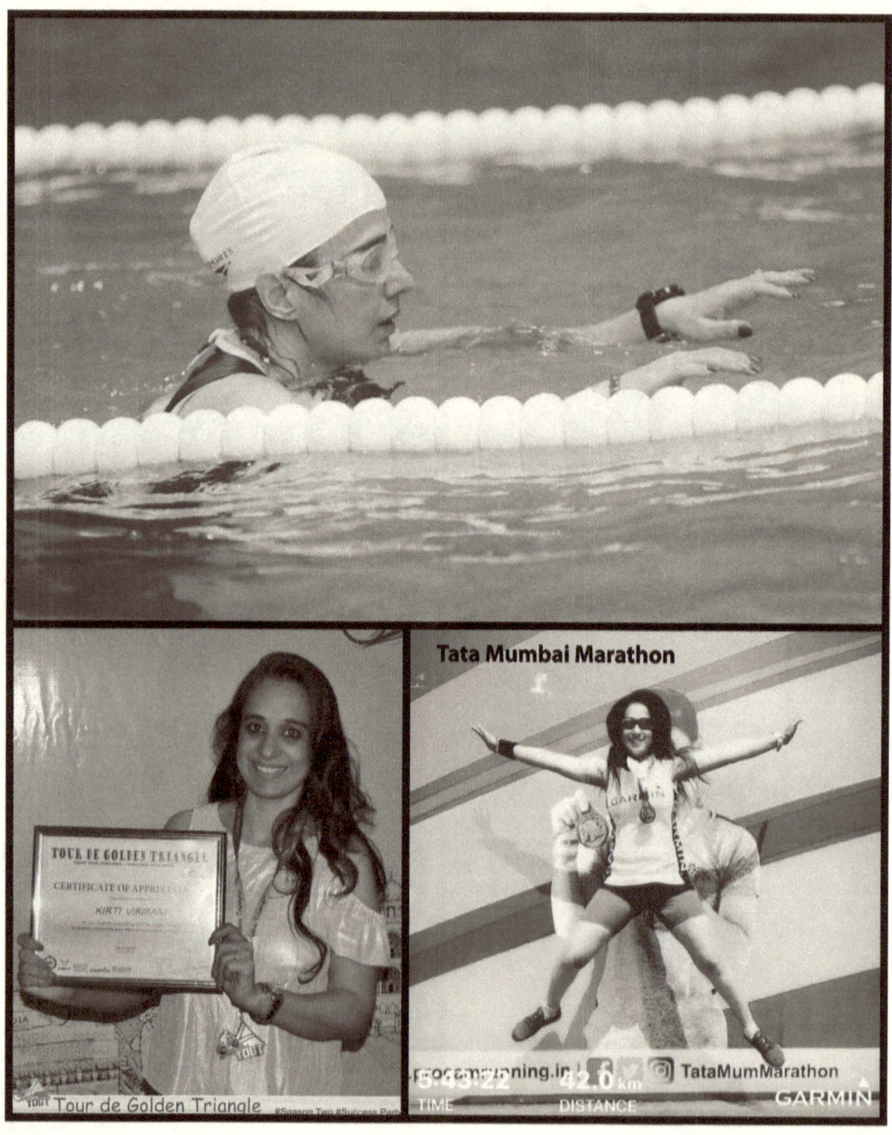
Tata Mumbai Marathon
Tour de Golden Triangle
TataMumMarathon
TIME
DISTANCE
GARMIN

A Podium Mother 02

Smithaa Kajale, Mumbai

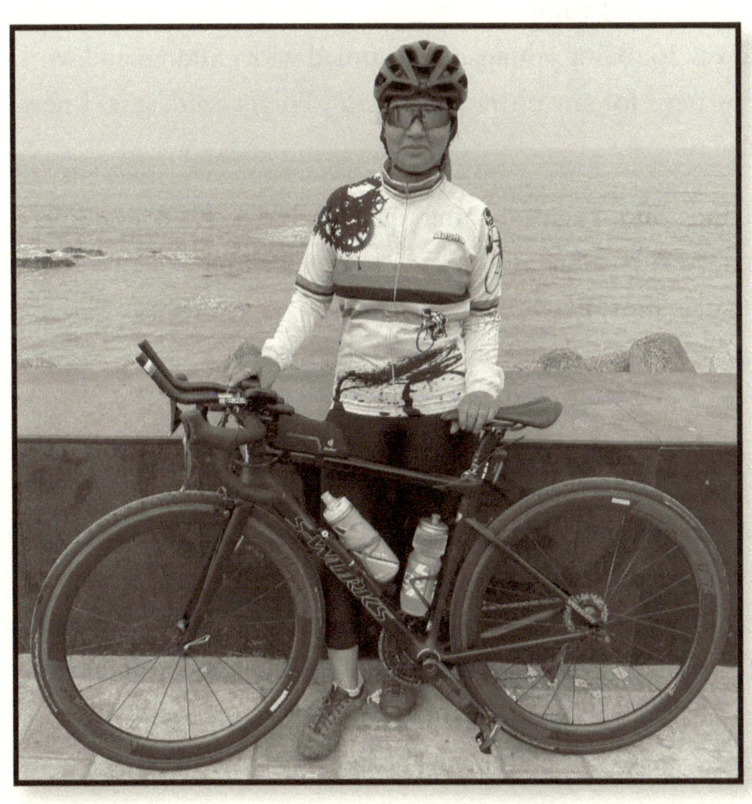

A civil engineer by profession, winner of several cycling races, third rank holder at Kolhapur Triathlon 2019, second rank holder at Nagpur Triathlon 2020, National qualifier at Nashik Association Championship 2020; a 45-year-old with troubled menopause, yet a winner, this is Smithaa Kajale from Thane.

My Early Life

I was born in Kolkata, and my father was in the Indian Air Force. His last posting was in Nashik, after which, he retired and joined Hindustan Aeronautics Limited (HAL). I started studying civil engineering and soon, my parents decided to get me married as they did not want to let go of a suitable and desirable match.

I got married at the age of 18 and had my first child at 19. I continued with my education and completed my bachelor's. My second child was born when I was 26. Being young and occupied with children and work, I never felt the need for any physical workout. Forget exercising, I never even walked.

After my second child, I started going for short walks. Even a kilometer used to seem like a colossal task. Then, my husband and I decided to start with regular morning brisk walks. It was refreshing to walk and talk amidst all the house duties and busy schedules.

It Started as Casual Fitness

Fast forward to when my elder son turned 19. He started going to the gym. I followed his footsteps. I got into a habit of regular workout and weight training. When my younger son turned 17, he started outdoor cycling and gradually it became his passion. He started participating in races. He did MTB Nashik, Thane Cycling Championship, and in December 2017, he won a gold medal at the national time trial.

All it took for me to start cycling was a little coaxing and pushing from my younger son. He was sure that I would enjoy riding. I was getting bored of gymming. I usually get bored by routine; hence I bought a basic cycle and started cycling in December 2018.

In February 2019, I won the first prize at Navi Mumbai Maha Cyclothon and with it, a cash prize of Rs. 10,000. In March 2019, I won the 3rd prize in the open category at Pedal Cyclothon. In April 2019, I won the 3rd Prize in the open category at Borivali Cycling Association Time Trial. I started loving my finishes and the joy of winning. It is said that a child gives birth to a mother, and truly my children gave birth to a new me.

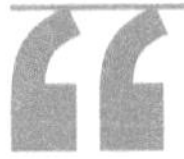

"The moment a child is born, the mother is also born. She never existed before. The woman existed, but the mother, never. A mother is something absolutely new."

Anonymous

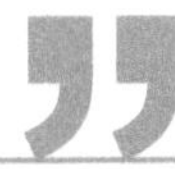

Take That Chance

Next, I heard about Triathlon from one of the members of my cycling group. The concept of Triathlon and the idea of participating were attractive and seemed exciting, but there was a problem – I had never run until now!

Soon, both my sons were going to be in the U.S. and so I would be free from their day-to-day responsibilities. Life in motherhood revolves around children, and they become our priority. I was no different. The empty nest syndrome was real, and I needed to distract myself.

I decided to take the plunge and try out this new excitement in my life-Triathlon. Under the guidance of Viv Menon for triathlon plans and Nimesh for swimming, I participated in the Kolhapur Triathlon (Olympic distance) and stood third. It was my first open water swim experience and I was kicked, smashed, punched all over due to the massive number of participants.

After Kolhapur, I thought of going back to cycling. Meanwhile, someone mentioned Tigerman Tri, Nagpur in Feb 2020. My previous doubts vanished, and I registered for the event. A week before the Tigerman event, I came across the Nashik Tri association championship. The championship was attractive, and after a discussion with my coach Viv, I registered for the event.

"Sometimes we have one chance to ride that wave,
one opportunity to jump on, take a deep breath and
feel the rush of adrenaline…don't miss your chance."

Heidi Reagan

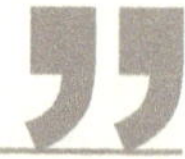

In February, I knew that Nashik would be cold, and I didn't have the wetsuit for the race. Hence I started going for early morning swims and bathing in cold water to acclimatize my body. I came to know the swim would be in the pool, and I took a sigh of relief.

When I collected my bib, I was informed that the swim would take place in a dam (water reservoir). I couldn't sleep for the entire night. The race morning was horrifying than the revelation of the previous eve. To my amazement, there were no ropes, buoys, or any emergency evacuation.

Upon questioning, the officials made it clear that the race was a time trial for the national qualifier and is a self-supported race. I took a while to register this fact. My throat went dry. In already cold weather, I stood there, shivering in a swimsuit. I prayed and chanted what I could remember and asked my husband to wait for me until I completed my swim and jumped in the water. I finished the 1500 meters swim course in 35 mins. After completing the bike course, which was an undulating path, and the run in the scoring heat, I stood fourth. A week after I participated in Tigerman Triathlon, Nagpur, and stood second.

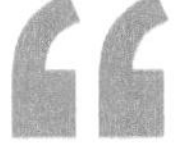

"Inaction breeds doubt and fear. Action breeds confidence and courage. If you want to conquer fear, do not sit home and think about it. Go out and get busy."

Dale Carnegie

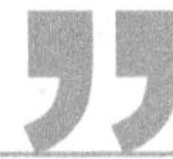

Menopause Havoc

For the event in November, I started training in June 2019. At the same time, I had to travel to Pennsylvania to meet my elder son. There, the issue of menopause started. I was continuously bleeding heavily for a week to 10 days and changing menstrual cups every hour. Without a country-specific prescription, I could not take any medications in the U.S., hence I continued in the same state until I returned to India.

I felt weak and lacked stamina. I consulted my physician as the race was nearing, and I had to get into vigorous training. My blood test reports were not at all satisfying. My hemoglobin was at 8. My physician strictly advised me not to attempt any race, which was just two months away.

"Do not attempt" doesn't go well with me, hence I asked for a solution. He advised an intravenous blood transfusion. I readily agreed and went to his clinic after work and got the I.V. It is common to get a fever after the I.V., and I got it too. My husband was concerned for me; he was always intrigued by this training idea and kept asking me, *"Kyun Kar Rahi ho?"* (Why are you doing this?).

I recovered the hemoglobin level, but my bleeding didn't stop. Thankfully, just ten days before the race day, God showed mercy on me, and I wasn't bleeding anymore. I could say one thing, *"Der aae durust aae."* (Something on the lines better late than never).

On the eve of the Kolhapur Tri, I went for the bike route recce with my husband, and I felt exhausted in just 2–3 km. I was anxious about the race the next day. I believe that the mind conspires to what you start thinking, I had made up my mind to finish the race, and I did. I concluded that from my menopause episode.

"Leaders bleed, period."

Silvia Young, My Fem Truth: Scandalous Survival Stories

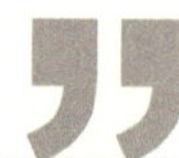

On to The Next

My boys are my pillars of strength. I haven't had any race where my husband wasn't there to cheer, support, and encourage me. My two boys were my initial coaches, guides, and mentors. I followed their footsteps in my workout/fitness journey as well as cycling.

I enrolled for Ironman 70.3 in Boulder, USA, but due to COVID, all the races got canceled. I will attempt the race whenever the racing season opens. I aim to continue on my fitness journey and emerge as a more vital human being mentally and physically.

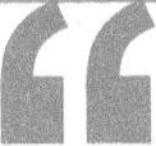

"A woman's health is her capital."

Harriet Beecher Stowe

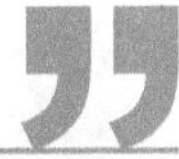

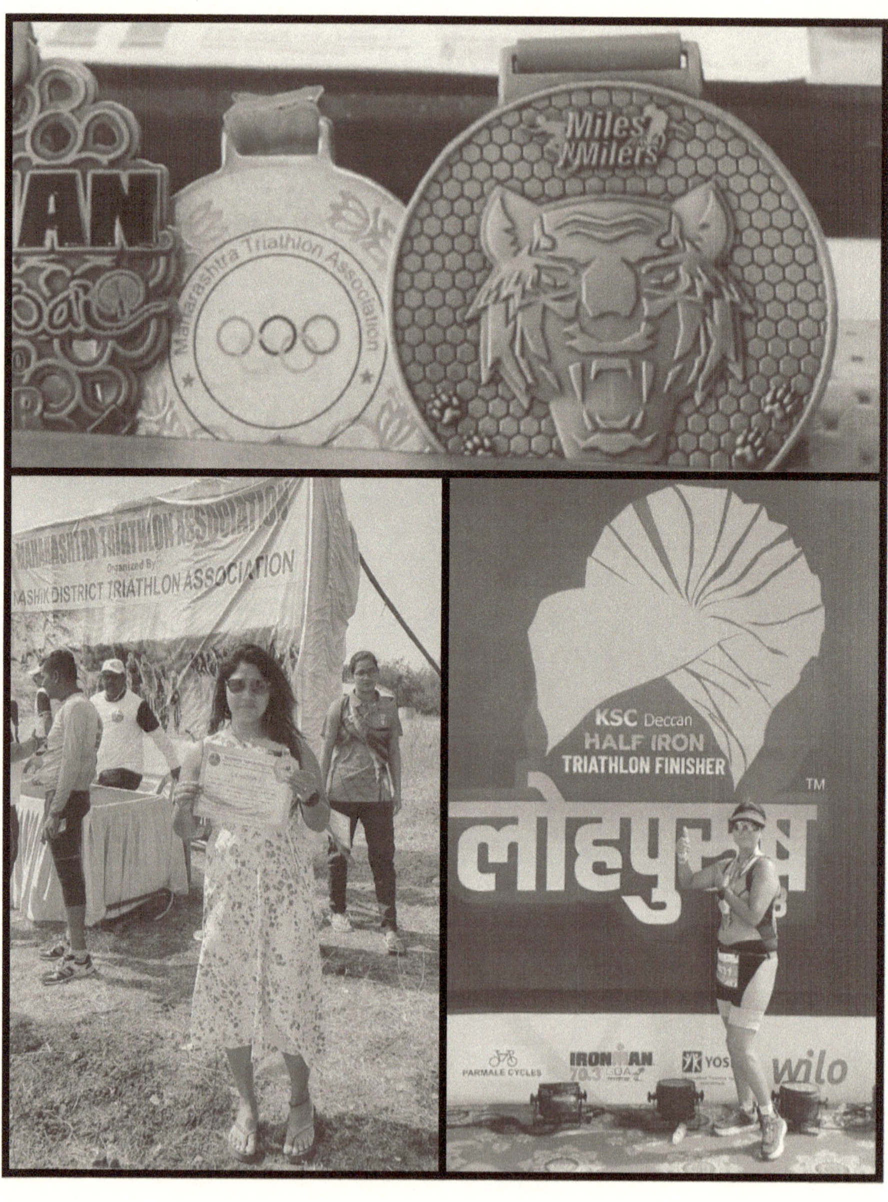
Miles
NMilers
Maharashtra Triathlon Association
MAHARASHTRA TRIATHLON ASSOCIATION
Organized By
NASHIK DISTRICT TRIATHLON ASSOCIATION
KSC Deccan
HALF IRON
TRIATHLON FINISHER
TM
लोहपुरुष
PARMALE CYCLES
IRONMAN
70.3
YOS
wilo

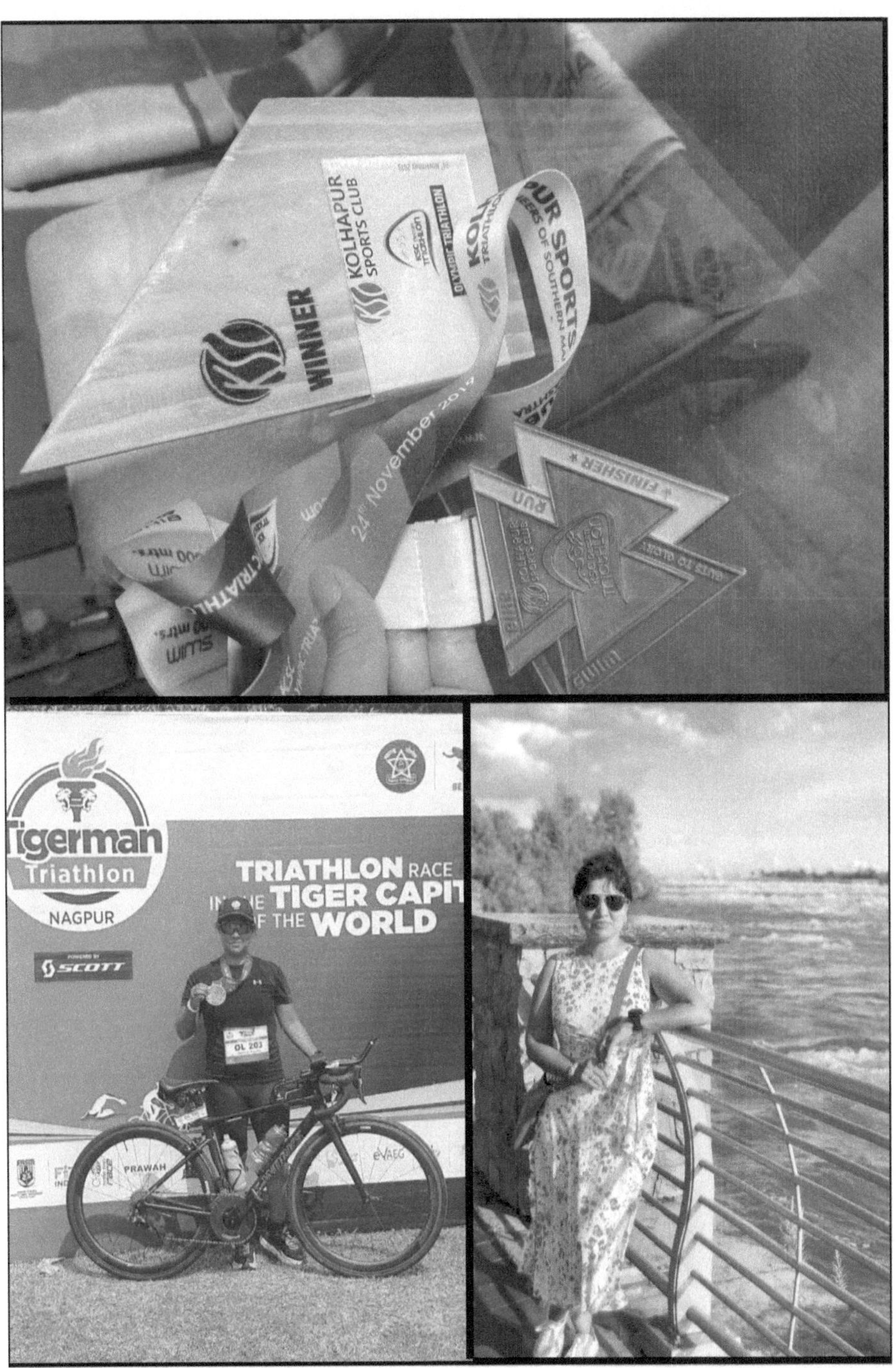

Especially Special   03

Deepa Katrodia

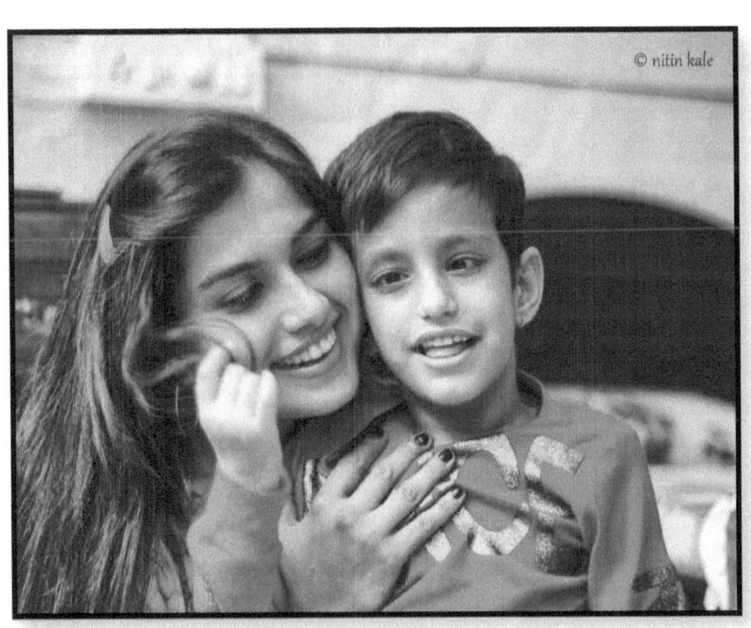

She got to hold her child's hand for a while, but she continues to hold her heart. First position Bangalore ultra 75K 2013, Winner Bangalore ultra 100K 2014, Finisher Hyderabad 70.3, Colombo 70.3, finisher at several half marathons, marathons and ultra runs, a fighter, giver, and above all a survivor in all aspects of life, a flawless Garba dancer, mother, and an excellent cook, this is 36-year-old Deepa from Mumbai.

Just a Girl Next Door

I was born in Indore in a joint Gujarati family. I am the youngest of three sisters. My birth took away the hope of having a boy in the family. My mother tells me that once I was brought home from the hospital, I became the apple of everyone's eye. My father who didn't even come to see me in the hospital would always cuddle and cradle me. I was too young to understand the law of attraction then, but I experienced that later in life. Eventually, my younger brother was born, and my family was "complete" now.

In Gujarati families, food is emotion, and that led to me piling on kilos. When the pleats of my skirt started widening, I understood that it's time to work hard on myself. As girls were not allowed to move out alone, I accompanied a neighbor on the morning walks. I didn't shed any weight, but I was happy walking as this was the only physical activity I had ever done.

I completed my bachelor's in commerce with no career goals at all. My only aim in life was to complete the necessary education and get married. Seeing the restrictions that come with living in small towns, my only condition for marrying was that I wanted to marry someone who lived in a city. In 2005, I married Pradeep and shifted to Mumbai.

Pradeep loved the outdoors. He was a regular trekker and went hiking in the Sahyadris around Mumbai. Like my other Gujarati friends and family members, once I got married, my world revolved around my partner. Pradeep's friends suggested he either dispose of his hiking boots or get his wife interested in hiking. He chose the latter.

Although we had a big family of eight members, and there were lots of house chores to be done, Pradeep was always understanding and supportive. I managed to take time off and went for shorter hikes with Pradeep. Later, we ended up doing the Gangotri trek together. In 2006 I gave birth to my daughter, Misri.

In Between Misri and My First Race

I had a normal pregnancy and a safe delivery. A few months after her birth, I started feeling that Misri's growing pattern was different. Assuming that a few children grow slowly as compared to others, I continued to enjoy my new motherhood. Pradeep found his life in Misri. Once I took her to Indore, and she suffered an injury, Pradeep suggested getting her to Mumbai for better treatment. The doctors recommended a few tests and then told us that Misri is suffering from "some" syndrome, which I didn't understand. We got a lot of tests done over three years to understand the disorder, in vain.

Misri was like an infant when she turned a year old. I used to cover and take her for the evening stroll lying to people about her age. People used to stare at us because we had a special child in our arms. We took her to Delhi, allowing the laboratories to send her sample to Japan for intense research to identify the disorder. I was also touted in a mall where a female saw us with Misri and assured us to give a herb that will cure her.

Desperation for our child made our mind numb and we were willing to try everything to find a cure. We followed that lady through a dark narrow lane and entered a small, shabby hut, Pradeep held me back and we left the place with Misri. Our hit and trial efforts continued with no results.

I started taking her to the physiotherapy center, where I came face to face with other children with different disorders. It was tough to absorb the fact, but it was high time we did it. We then took a call to accept that Misri is a unique child, and she'll need us lifelong. We were no longer hesitant in telling her real age or hid her when in public places. People's piercing eyes didn't bother us anymore.

Days were getting more challenging as Misri wouldn't sleep at all. I was awake 24*7 with significantly less sleep. Pradeep, my in-laws, and I worked as a team around Misri and took turns to sleep, but it wasn't enough. Pradeep would rock her the entire night. We were mentally exhausted, and there was a visible discord between us.

Both of us consciously took a call to devote time to ourselves and stay healthy to take care of Misri. With the change in medication, Misri started sleeping for a while in the morning. Pradeep and I began our regular morning walks in Borivali National Park. My in-laws pitched in and offered to take care of Misri in our absence. Our slow walks turned into jogs and finally into faster runs as we had just one hour for ourselves when Misri slept.

The caretaker at the physiotherapy center suggested that I participate in the dream run. I was always fascinated by the Mumbai Marathon whenever I watched the race on the television. Pradeep got the half marathon form in July for himself, and because he wasn't sure about my training, he suggested that I should participate in the dream run. I was baffled at the thought to run amidst strangers and asked him to register me for the half marathon as well.

The biggest issue was – who was going to l take care of Misri in our absence? My mother-in-law offered full support and encouraged us to run. We trained together for six to seven months, one hour every day. I crossed the finish line of the first half marathon in two hours and

13 minutes holding Pradeep's hand. In July 2012, four months after the half marathon, I registered for a full marathon.

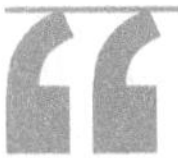

First is always special. A girl who had no aim in life to a mother whose only purpose now was to be there in a fit and healthy state for her daughter. The finish line gave meaning to my life.

Run, for My Daughter Will Never Be Able to Do So

We then joined the Nike running club and slowly graduated in learning the running terminology along with new terms and conditions about Misri's health. In 2013, I crossed the finish line of the 42.2 km full marathon along with Pradeep, in four hours and 49 minutes.

I wanted to run longer now. Someone told me about ultra runs. I was attracted by the distance. Pradeep was not keen and asked me to train and that he would take care of Misri. I took a yearly plan from Daniel Vaz, a marathon coach, and started with religious training. We flew to Bangalore, and Pradeep stayed with Misri in the hotel room while I went ahead to the start line of my first 75 km Bangalore Ultra Marathon.

I finished the run in 11 hours and 43 minutes, stood at the podium, while Pradeep cheered for me at the finish line with Misri. Misri's condition continued to deteriorate with each passing day. We learned something new with every new symptom. Meanwhile, I continued running.

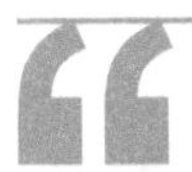

Running gave me a lot of self-confidence and strength to dedicate to Misri. Everyone in the family stood by each other as the most robust support.

After the 75 km Ultra Marathon, I was keen to do a 100 km run. Pradeep registered for a 75 km Ultra, and both of us started our training under the guidance of Daniel Vaz. This time, both of us were running hence taking Misri along was not possible. My mother and mother-in-law offered to take care of Misri, which made us feel relaxed for the run.

I started the race at a turtle's pace as I was keen to finish rather than messing up. At the 75th km mark, I observed some cheering at the podium, and when I craned my neck, I saw Pradeep conquering the podium. I was thrilled to the core, and then something happened, my feet just started rolling, my pace increased substantially. I finished the race in 17 hours.

I never bought any shoes for Misri for I knew that my child would never be able to walk or run, she would never address us as Papa and Mamma. So, we ran the distances for Misri, we compensated for her falling and learning to walk.

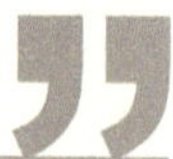

The Tri Game

In between training for marathons, Pradeep was keenly following triathlon videos and tri-athletes. He started to learn swimming. He registered for the Chennai Triathlon and got a road bike worth 52 thousand for training. We had to keep the bike cost a secret as we knew we would not be able to justify the expense.

I used to cycle on a basic bike. One day I took Pradeep's bike and rode from Malad to Borivali. That day I realized why my neck and back used to hurt while I rode my bike. But buying one more new bike was out of the question. Our primary focus was on Misri's treatment, so managing expenses was critical. Both of us were preparing for the same event, but buying the accessories in pairs was difficult. We managed all the things in between us and started training alternately.

Misri's condition continued to deteriorate. She didn't open her eyes or respond. But we continued to share all our racing and training stories with her. After Pradeep's successful completion of the Chennai Triathlon, I also started to learn swimming. I had to unlearn and start afresh. I used to mimic the swimming stance throughout the day. I registered for the Chennai Tri, but the event got canceled. We then registered for the Pune Triathlon. Our close friend came to assist Misri while both Pradeep and I went for the race.

I was scared of open water and didn't step into the lake. I was just a mere spectator. I felt sorry and disgusted with myself and grateful for all the help that poured in to enable us to participate in the race. Later, I completed the first Olympic Distance Triathlon in Kolhapur. I started loving the sport and the thrill to train for three different sports was marvelous.

Pradeep went ahead and finished his comrades. Being an expensive race, I stayed back with Misri while he came back with a bronze medal and we proudly dangled it around Misri's neck. Misri was not showing any signs of improvement, and it was tough for us to accept the reality. Keeping all odds at bay, we started training for the Hyderabad Ironman 70.3, 2017 together.

Even though we got Misri's flight ticket to Hyderabad, we decided to let her stay at home due to overexertion while we headed for our race. Both of us completed the race. I crossed the finish line in eight hours and thirty-two minutes. While boarding the flight back, I felt an uncomfortable stomach-churning. I called up home to ask about Misri, and my mother gave a satisfactory answer. The uneasiness continued all through the journey. Once we reached home, Misri was running a high fever. Upon consultation, the doctor prescribed some medicine. We fed Misri and went to bed.

It was a regular practice for me to check Misri's heartbeat whenever she slept. That was the only way to check her existence, as otherwise, she won't respond for hours. That night I couldn't feel her heartbeat.

When Pradeep and I held her in our arms, she looked at us and then closed her eyes forever. All of a sudden, the house turned silent. Our life revolved around Misri, and it appeared as if we had nothing to do anymore. The chaos of time management, the rush for doctor's appointments, the sleepless nights, everything came to a standstill.

Pradeep was shattered. He stopped his training even when he had to race for a full Ironman Malaysia in 15 days. He was not ready to participate. He was mentally disturbed as Misri was his heart and soul. With lots of encouragement and counseling, we went together for his race. He finished the race in 13 hours and 14 minutes. He was among the top 10 Indians to finish the race and received a sponsored participation for Malaysia 70.3 the next year.

He was not keen to participate, hence he asked me to race. I worked on all three sports, especially the swim. I crossed the finish line at the Malaysia 70.3, 2018 in 7 hours and 42 minutes. In 2019, I also participated in TFN (Tour of Nilgiris) and stood 10th in the female category.

Do It for Yourself; No One Else Will Do It for You

We never had outside help for Misri. All of us worked like an F-1 race team – prompt, accurate, and knowing our jobs well. Our life was nothing beyond Misri and racing. Now that the central element was missing there was a vacuum in our life. Pradeep had to get back to his job while I was still trying to figure out my way. I always loved to dance; hence I did Zumba certification. I also got certified as a Reebok fitness trainer. I started taking Zumba sessions in three schools and loved my stint. I was dancing my heart out and also interacting with children. I used to see Misri in all of them.

Pradeep and I got associated with organizations that work for children with special needs. During Navratri 2020, both of us organized a fundraiser for one such organization by cycling 90 km for 9 days. With our experience, we know the expense incurred in the treatment, and the mental trauma parents go through. It is our small gesture to help many parents and children.

Pradeep and I worked hard on ourselves to bear as well as come out of our massive loss. Any medal, podium, or finish line is dedicated to our daughter Misri who could never express her emotions, but we as parents understood whatever she said. We know she is happy to see us racing and finishing.

We shall continue to race and cover distances for our daughter, who never even stood on her own feet.

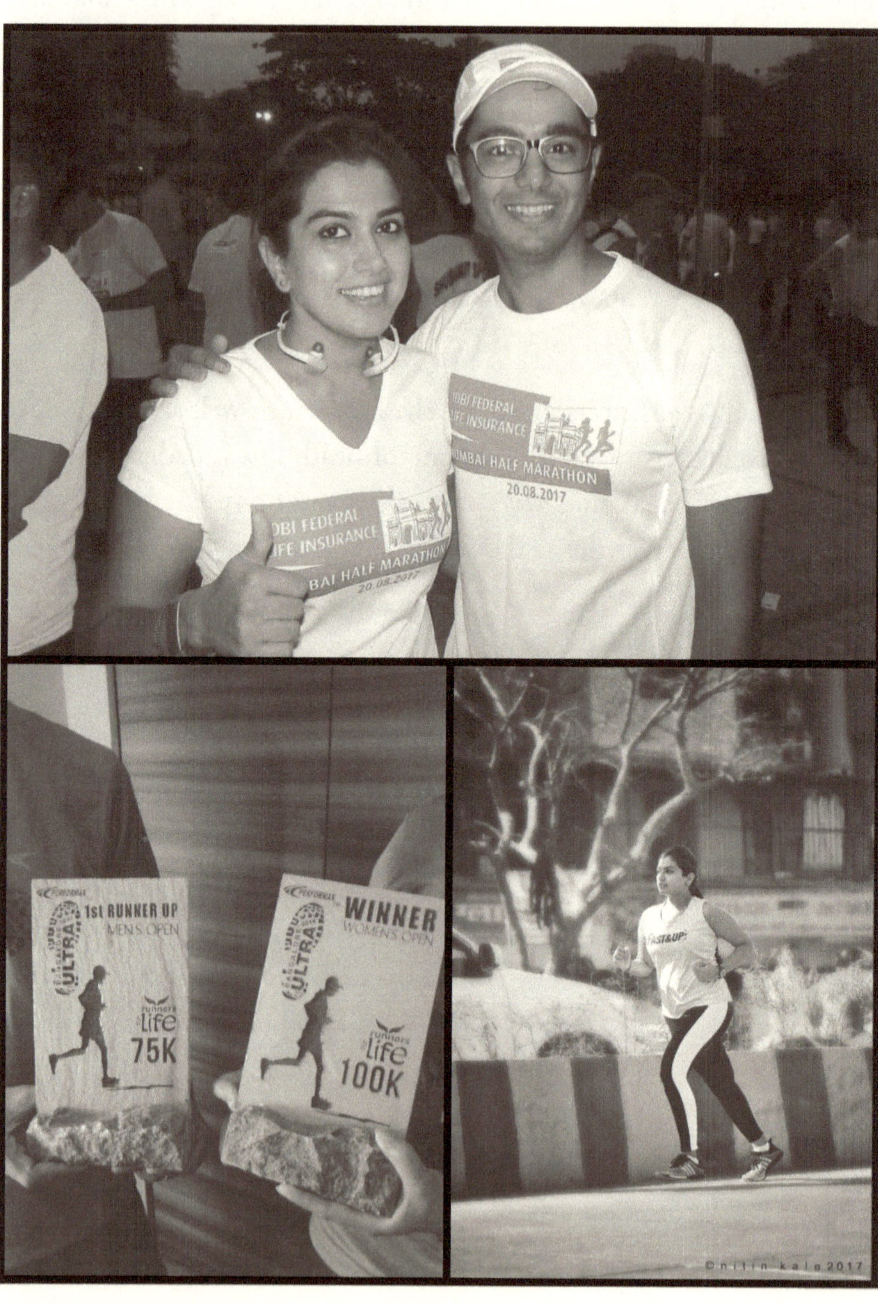
IDBI FEDERAL
LIFE INSURANCE
MUMBAI HALF MARATHON
20.08.2017
IDBI FEDERAL
LIFE INSURANCE
MUMBAI HALF MARATHON
20.08.2017
1st RUNNER UP
MEN'S OPEN
ULTRA
runners
Life
75K
WINNER
WOMEN'S OPEN
ULTRA
runners
Life
100K
FAST&UP
©nitin kale 2017

4:15 HR. Pacer
4:45 HR. Pacer
5:00 HR. Pacer
5:30 HR. Pacer

skechers
GOrun
Reliance Trends
TimingTechnologies
1
2
3

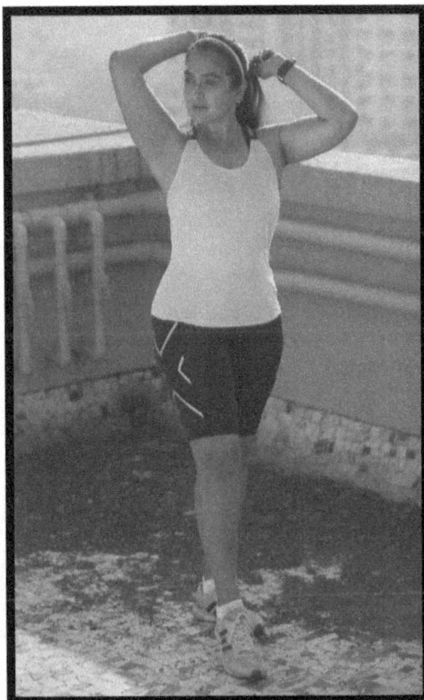

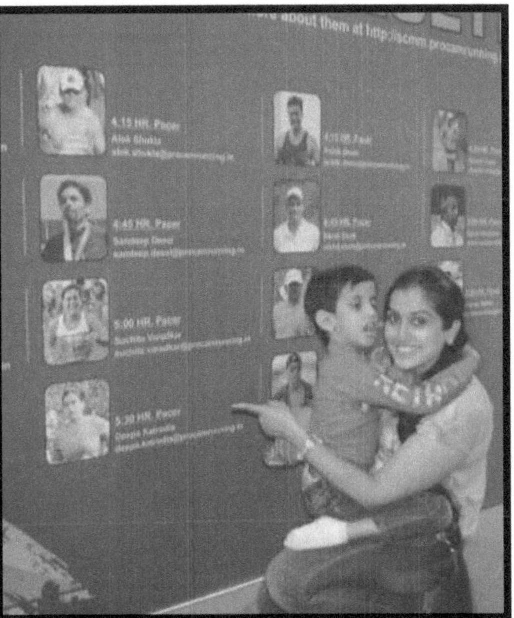

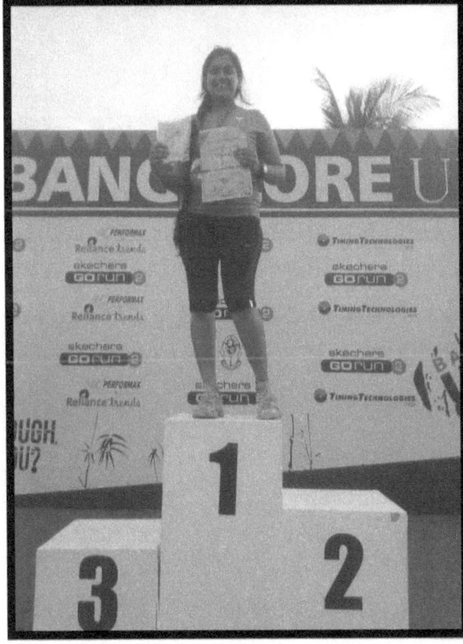

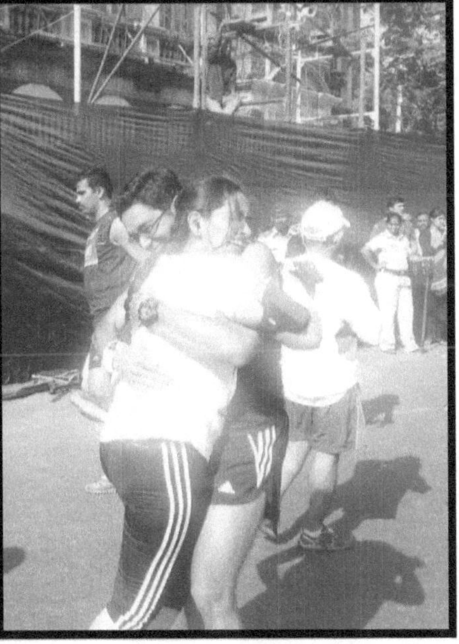

Every Finish Line is a New Beginning | 04

If There is Darkness Then There is a Finish Line Too; Tenacity of a Rock

Parul Sheth, Mumbai

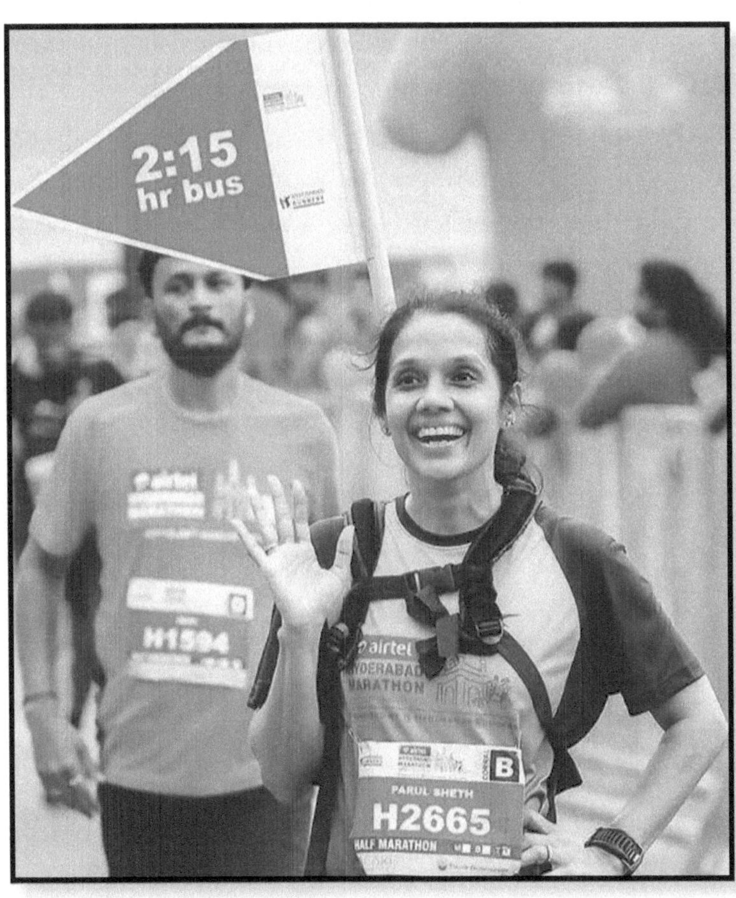

An architect by profession and also of her life, a fast runner and a furious chaser of the finish line, Boston marathoner, pacer at Mumbai Marathon, finisher of Dubai Ironman 70.3, author of an inspirational book – *"A running soul"*, an entrepreneur, mother of two, here is 48-year-old, a woman of substance, filled with positivity with a beautiful smile, Parul Sheth from Mumbai.

An Easy-Breezy Childhood

I was born in Mumbai and lived in a big joint family. I was the firstborn of the family, hence was treated like an angel and enjoyed all the pampering— a few of the memorable treasures of my childhood. I have always been an easy-going person; never pushed myself for anything. I took things as they came. I was above average in sports but wasn't the athlete kind. Back then, the pressure to attend any sport or skill-building class was not a standard affair; hence, I didn't have sports training of any type. After finishing a bachelor's degree in science, I realized that I didn't have the tenacity to be a doctor hence shifted to architecture.

I then got married and continued to work as before. I was a fit person. I got my active genes from my parents. I continued going to the gym and kept myself fit. Life was easy and straightforward.

The U-Turn

My life was going on. I was a mother of two kids now, and like any other moms, was juggling, managing, running errands between work, children, and home. I had my hands full of responsibilities.

Then, 2003 came as a big shock.

I faced the untimely demise of my husband. Due to this sudden loss, my world came to a standstill. I felt lost and disoriented. From shared responsibilities, I was now on my own. I had to manage everything on my own including two young children. My family and friends came in as tremendous support. But I believe that no one can fight a battle for you; one has to stand at the forefront and face the shelling.

I had to get back on track and bring my life back to normal as my kids were my major responsibility. I had to push myself out of the dungeon. In 2005, my friends made me register for the Mumbai Marathon. They told me it was like a big party on Mumbai's streets and everyone was excited about it. The primary reason was that they wanted me to move out of the house. I trained for it on my own. As I ran, I felt the lightness in my head, decluttering of thoughts and freedom from the darkness.

The training ran in parallel with my healing process. I surrendered myself to my pulsating heartbeat and the heavy breath while running.

In 2005, I finished my first half marathon with a strong stride. The finish line made me a stronger person. I was releasing my anxiousness with every drop of sweat. I was tougher than I thought, faster than I realized, and a winner that I never imagined. There was no looking back from here. I just wanted to move ahead with a strong vision.

Aim Big, Always

I found my flights of fantasy in running. I finished a few half marathons. My running became stronger with lots of training and hard work. I now wanted to graduate to full marathons, but my speed (in comparison to my running buddies), was still an issue. I wanted to finish my marathon in good timing and strongly. I always wondered, and asked my fellow running buddies – how they ran fast?

I was working hard, but somehow, I felt that I wasn't pushing myself enough. Everyone was talking about pace, finish timing and many such jargons, which were foreign to me. I asked my friend, "What do you mean by running fast?"

Sandeep knew my hustle and told me reassuringly, "I'll help." Until then, I had been a non-Garmin runner, but then he instructed me to get into structured running and have a Garmin for proper tracking. Training plans were made, and I started my training for a 5k, 10K, time interval, threshold and zone running. I was trying to fit myself into the world of daunting training plans. I also owe Savio big time for he made me a runner. He truly pushed me hard. It helped me in moving my darkness behind.

In 2012, with all the discipline, I ran my first marathon in 4:35 hours. In 2014, a day before the SCMM race, I wanted to relax and was searching for a movie online. Back then, content was not so readily available, and someone suggested watching "The Marathon". After the movie, I kept wondering what was the Boston Marathon all about.

Google gave me information that kept me in awe of the race. The Boston Marathon is an annual marathon race hosted by several cities in greater Boston in eastern Massachusetts, United States. The Boston Marathon is the world's oldest annual marathon and ranks as one of the world's best road racing events. It is one of six World Marathon Majors.

The Boston Marathon is open to runners 18 years or older from any nation, but they must meet certain qualifying standards. The qualifying criterion is based on age and gender and to enter the race it is mandatory to finish the qualifying race in three hours and fifty minutes or less.

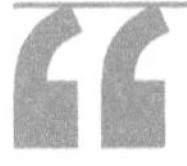

> *"The human body has limitations; the human spirit is boundless."*
>
> ### *Dean Karnazes*

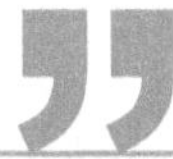

At the age of 42, I was a four hours and 30 minutes runner, and pushing below four hours would be a herculean task. Boston was my dream now, and I was eager to stand at the start line of the prestigious race. I dedicated myself totally to the training and sincerely followed the plans. Then after three years of not-a-single-day-missing training, at the age of 45, I finished the qualifying race, the Rotterdam marathon in three hours and forty-eight minutes! I was officially Boston-qualified.

I flew to Boston with lots of anxiety, tension and butterflies in my tummy. Savio wasn't just being my running coach but a mentor as well. He read my mind and asked me to relax and run. I took a deep breath, carried a broad smile, held my head high and ran with all my might to finish the Boston marathon in four hours and two minutes. Once I finished the Boston Marathon, I had no further urge to get faster. After all, I wondered what I could do faster than this? So, I continued to enjoy running and training at a similar pace.

I had a deep desire to give back to my city, Mumbai. A city that stood by me through thick and thin, a city that gave me wings to fly, a city where I touched my first finish line. I wanted that many should strongly finish their marathon, many should be able to get their PB, for you never know who is chasing the finish line with what background. At the start line, we all stand united, each one of us has a different aspiration to run a marathon, but we run with a common goal to reach the finish line with pride. In 2018, I paced the Mumbai marathon for a 4.30 hours bus.

What Next?

I was satisfied and happy with my running, and with no further wish to get faster, I wondered what next? In 2018 someone in the group suggested registering for Goa Triathlon. As a part of my Boston training, I used to swim a little, but that was it. I was indeed not ready for a race. The closing date for the registration was coming closer, and the 500 rupee discount was also getting over (so cheesy) so along with a few friends I registered for the Goa Triathlon Olympic Distance.

I could barely swim one lap – 23 meters in a pool, and I didn't have a bike yet I was attempting the Triathlon that's the level of risk-taking capacity I own. My friend Russa offered to swim next to me, and I sighed with relief. I then borrowed a bike and finished the Triathlon in sub 4. (well! I think that's my favorite figure) There is always an itch to go after higher goals, and I never wanted to stop at the Olympic distance hence I registered for Dubai 70.3.

Under the experienced guidance of Ashutosh Barve, I worked to improve my swimming, which is still a challenge. Viv gave me arduous but attainable training plans, and he made me reach the finish line. The triathlons made me explore myself. The combination of three sports to be finished within a time frame ensures that we grow on mental toughness as well and not just physical. It's a continuous journey of self-discovery.

Sooner or Later Doesn't matter, Start

I woke up to realize my strength later in life. I ran my first half marathon, SCMM in 2005. I ran my first full marathon, SCMM in 2012. I did my first Ironman 70.3 in 2019. I ran the Boston marathon after 14 years of my running journey.

During my Sunday long runs, whenever I am returning from Shivaji Park, which is at the 14th–15th km, I am always at my runner's high. It is at this moment that I feel I can attain anything. I start believing that I am a superhero. I make the most robust, as well as most stupid decisions during my runner's high feeling. I always need a good 14 km as a warm-up, then after my body goes with the flow and my feet follow the rhythm.

The way we say, Rome was not built in a day, similarly, the body needs time. One has to be consistent and keep putting in the effort day after day. It is crucial to building the endurance base; speed will eventually follow. I am a traditional runner who runs without a phone or music plugged in. I run and train with like-minded people who motivate and lift each other every moment.

Nature is our best teacher.

If there is a storm, then there will be calmness as well.

If there is darkness, then bright light will follow soon.

If there are mountains to climb, then there are rivers to swim, too.

If you can walk, then you can indeed run too

Get up.

Start

And see you at the finish line.

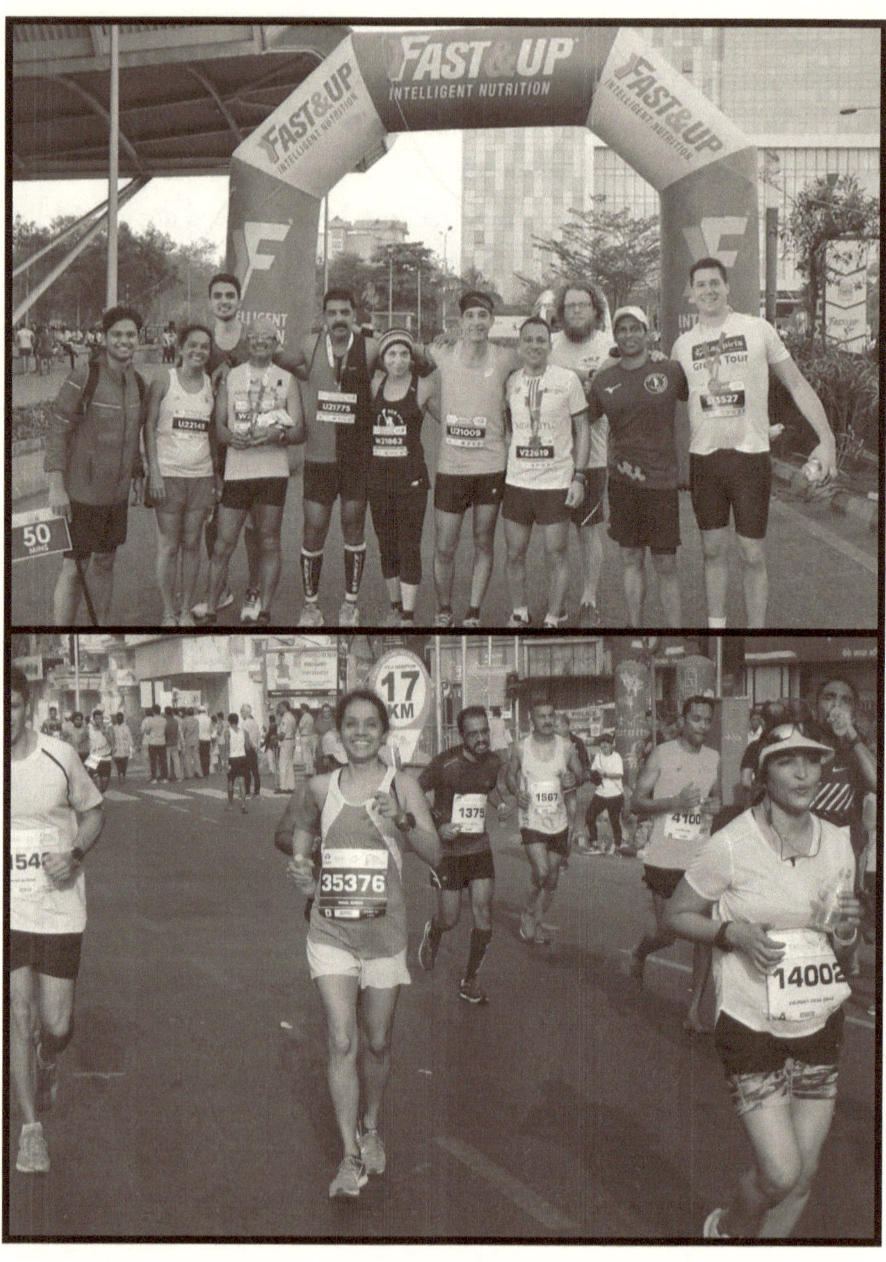

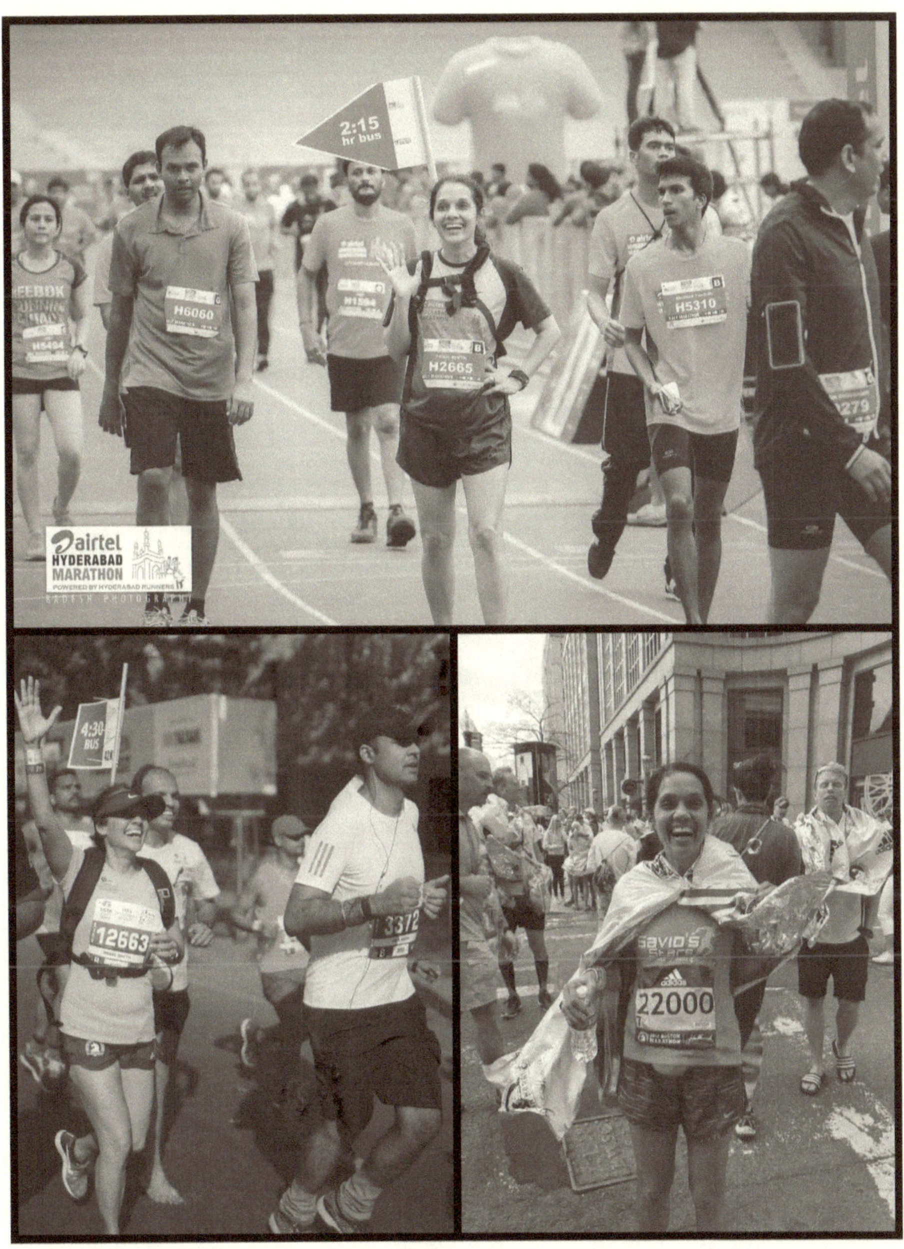

2:15
hr bus
H6060
H2665
H5310
4:30
BUS
12663
22000
airtel
HYDERABAD
MARATHON
POWERED BY HYDERABAD RUNNERS

Wake Up and Run | **05**

Super Sonic

Ketaki, Mumbai

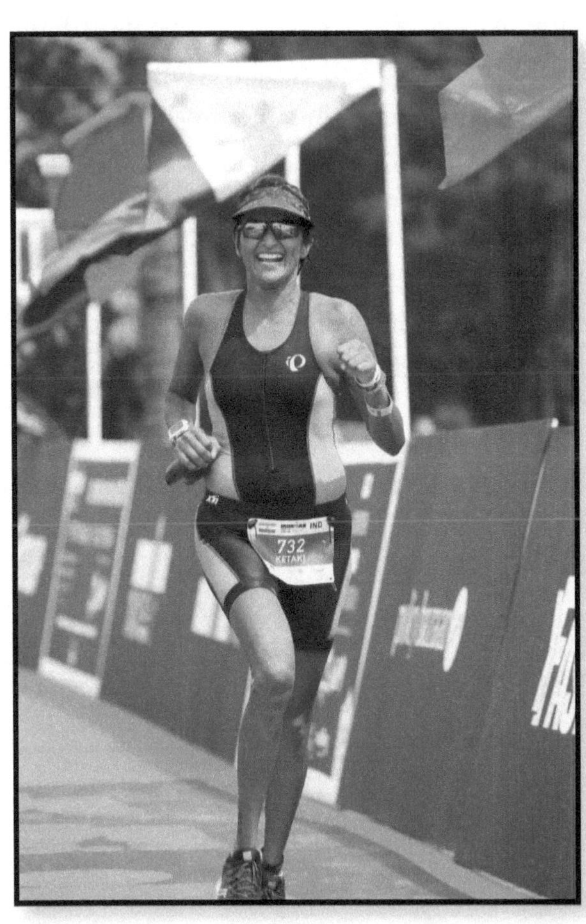

Squeezing in time for a run late in the night after her family was asleep and running in circles in her child's school playground while waiting for the school to end – 43-year-old Ketaki Agtey makes it clear – 'If she wants it, she'll go get it'. First Indian female finisher and second in her age category at Ironman Goa 70.3, first rank in Tigerman (Olympic distance) Triathlon 2020, second in age category in SCMM 2017, second in AG, Navi Mumbai HM 2017, a fauji kid, a PR and Communications professional, mother of two, Mumbai-based Ketaki shares her exciting stories.

My Outdoorsy Childhood

We are blessed to be born to this fabulous couple who raised my sister and me to be independent, fierce and sensitive human beings. Growing up, we were an outdoorsy, adventurous and fun-loving family. I have traveled a fair bit and lived in places like Iraq, Wellington and Gorakhpur, among others.

I was into athletics during my school days and have grown up rough and tough. The love for the outdoors runs in the family. Whilst in Iraq, we made a road trip from Baghdad to London and back with a four-person tent on the carrier of the car et al…!

We were raised in an environment agnostic to gender, religion, caste, creed, etc. Equality, partnership and respect for another human being was of prime importance. One of the main mantras to live by was, 'work is worship' and 'always have the courage of conviction.'

I did most of my schooling and college in the garden city, Bangalore, and started my career in Public Relations there.

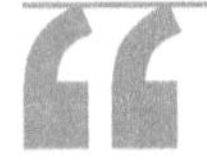

"Call it a clan, call it a network, call it a tribe, call it a family. Whatever you call it, whoever you are, you need one."

Jane Howard

Catch Me If You Can

I got married in 2000 and shifted to the US for a while and that's where my running journey began, including the love for outdoor running. We then moved back to Mumbai, and by then, I was running 5–8 km thrice a week. In 2003, as part of regular annual medicals, I was diagnosed with hyperthyroidism. This autoimmune disease continues to be part of my daily existence, which I manage with medication. I do believe my active lifestyle has helped with managing a lot of the known side effects.

In 2004, I had my first child and within six weeks of my delivery, I got back to exercise and short runs. I was pleasantly surprised to see my body respond to physical activity by readjusting and shedding my pregnancy weight. I have always been lean and in the general average percentile of weight for my height and frame, so weight loss was not my target, but I aimed to build my stamina and work on the lost strength.

In 2009, my second child was born, and now it was challenging to manage work, children, schedules and other chores. There were days when I used to start my workout at 9.30 pm after putting my kids to sleep and wrapping up tasks.

The constant time management and juggling were getting tougher, hence I invested in a semi-commercial (full size, the type that is used in gyms – pulled out the stops on this one) treadmill at home, and thereby tried to eliminate excuses for missed runs.

The pounding on the treadmill became a lullaby to my kids. Despite having adequate resources, I was missing a certain sense of rhythm as I seemed to be tailoring my fitness activities around everyone else's schedules rather than prioritize them as a part of the whole. And thus began my journey of outdoor running 2.0 with renewed vigor and the purpose of prioritizing my fitness goals.

Along the way, I joined striders in 2013. Joining this dynamic and well-organized group was a fantastic decision! I came across like-minded people, and in the process, have made friends for life. Our conversations went beyond our professions and social status. I learned a lot about the nitty-gritty of running. I explored, read and became aware of the nuances of running, injury, recovery, types of shoes and much more. It opened a window to the world of endurance sport and ignited a passion that had been dormant thus far.

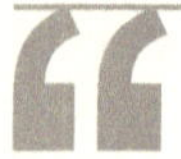

"I've learned through the years that it's not where you live, it's the people who surround you that make you feel at home."

J.B. McGee

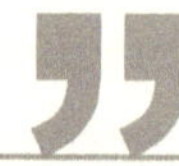

Gradually I started racing half marathons. I set myself a personal goal of doing a comfortable Sub-2 HM before taking the plunge into full marathons. Among the races I did over the years, some included the HM (Half Marathon) in Satara, HM in Amsterdam, several local and domestic runs including HTHM (Hiranandani Thane Half Marathon) and Powai runs. I also stood second in my age category in SCMM 2017. Receiving a podium medal at one of the most iconic marathons in the country was an exhilarating feeling! The fun cherry on the cake was a cash prize.

The journey for the fulls began with the first one being one of the BIG 5: Chicago Marathon. And then the personal goal of doing a sub 4 FM happened in the beautiful city of Riga, Latvia. My gift to myself for my 40th Birthday. (sub 4 means completing a full marathon 42.2 km under 4 hours)

Most recently, at the Hiranandani Thane Half Marathon 2020, I stood fourth in the women's open category, and I felt pride as the podium finishers were competitive athletes, all in their 20s. Felt chuffed at being somewhere near in their league.

Running is my happy space, and I can run in most weather conditions. Whenever I am unable to stick to the regular schedule, I complete my runs at any time of day even if it's slap bang in the middle of a hot and humid afternoon. Come heat, rain, shine or snow, I endeavor to always complete that scheduled run. I would like to say that I am always cautious and do take adequate measures when running at odd hours, be it additional hydration, running on shady routes, keeping someone in the know of my whereabouts, etc.

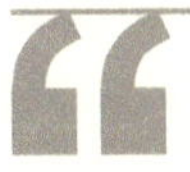

"Running is alone time that lets my brain unspool the tangles that build up over days. I run, pound it out on the pavement, channel that energy into my legs, and when I'm done with my run, I'm done with it."

Rob Haneisen

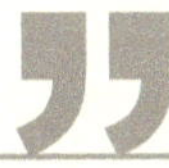

My Tryst with Cycling

I was advised to cut back (and ideally stop for a short period) on my running when I suffered shin splints and a stress fracture back in 2014. And so, in order to keep up with the cardio fitness, I went ahead and bought myself a hybrid bike. And thus began my tryst with cycling albeit the focus continued to be running.

2017 saw me going through various transitions across different aspects of my life. It is also the year I serendipitously stumbled into Triathlons. As they say – there is a time and place for everything, and it couldn't have been better timing for me to step into this amazing endurance sport. The very nature of my training changed. There was cycling and swimming now, in addition to running. This also meant fewer outdoor running days and more workouts throughout the week. The tempo and rhythm of the beast ensured high adrenaline levels to say the least!

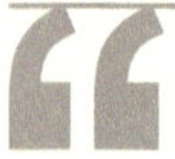

"Endurance is one of the most difficult disciplines, but it is to the one who endures that the final victory comes."

Gautam Buddha

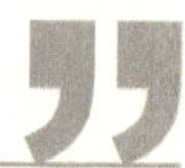

During that year (2017), I registered for the Kolhapur Triathlon, which was going to be my first Tri. Just two months before the race I'd graduated to cleats, and as part of the customary falls, I fractured my rib when the handlebar hit my chest. Thankfully I recovered before the race and went ahead to participate.

My first ever Triathlon was exciting and nerve-wracking, all at the same time. Being my first time in the open waters in India and being mortally terrified of the ecosystem in the cobalt blue-emerald waters of Rajaram Talav of Kolhapur, I was one of the last ones to finish the swim and that too doing the backstroke. I did, however, make up for the lost time on the bike and run leg and successfully finished my first Triathlon. Always a special one. The swim has and continues to be the weakest link, and I continue to work on it.

I started 2018 with the customary SCMM – Standard Chartered Mumbai Marathon (this year it became TMM – Tata Mumbai Marathon) and moved on to do the Goa Tri in February. As learning from my Kolhapur Tri, I'd decided to enroll for a swim camp in Goa in preparation towards my upcoming Goa Olympic Tri. I attended a swimming camp organized by coach Kaustubh Radkar. The learnings were invaluable. Albeit my swim time still left a lot to be desired, I completed the swim leg of the Goa Tri with ease and comfort.

The mountains beckoned in September 2018. Ladakh Marathon, a race that'd been on my wish list for a few years now, finally happened. The most breathtaking and beautiful race. Never have I been so tuned into my breath and HR (Heart Rate), as I was during this race. I came second in the Women's Open category.

I also did the Tour of Nilgiris (TFN) in December 2018. Although Nilgiris and the southern states are familiar ground, traversing these roads on a cycle was a rediscovery. TFN was a phenomenal experience. I came out as a more confident rider with better bike handling skills. This particular year at TFN (2018) saw the maximum number of women participants, both from India and abroad. It was wonderful to meet and interact with some high-performing endurance athletes. Needless to say, some lovely friendships were forged.

As the Tri journey continued, I felt it necessary to attack and build on all three disciplines (swim, bike and run) individually as well to perform better from an overall perspective. Before the Ironman Goa 70.3, I did the Goa swimathon in 2019. With some expert advice and guidance by star swimmer Nisha Madgavkar, the nervousness of open water swimming reduced tremendously. Little tips on calming down, treading the water, etc., did the trick. Open water panic is quite common, and it's been reported that even the most seasoned triathletes have panic attacks sometimes. Guidance, technique and practice helps in managing and overcoming the fear.

I would recommend attending open swim camps as a to-do to anyone signing up for an Ironman race. It would help to make you comfortable and confident about the swim.

Through my podium finish at the IM 70.3, Goa, I got a direct qualification to the Ironman 70.3 World Championships, to be held in Taupo NZ in November 2020. But alas! COVID-19 had different plans for us. I am scheduled to participate in the same in December 2022 and can't wait.

Children. Work. Home. Training. Repeat.

I try not to compromise on the essential parts of my life: my home life, my work life and my athlete life. It's quite the juggling act, but that's what makes it fun. My family knows that weekends are mum's heavy-duty training days; be it a long ride or long run or both. I get post-it notes on the bike or dining table wishing me a "good ride". The cherry on life's cake. It's such an uplifting feeling reading those surprise post-it notes just before heading out in the wee hours of a weekend morning.

A fun anecdote that any mum will relate to… the art of jugglery and masterful planning. Because we want our cake and want to eat it too! Non-negotiable 10K TT (Time Trials) meets non-negotiable early morning drop off for my child's overnight school trip. And so, permissions were sought, and I ran my 10K TT in the school ground post drop-off. Cut to my other child, casually walking up to class and musing at the "crazy person running circles in the school ground" until she realizes, much to her horror, who it was. She quickly skedaddled from the scene lest she had to admit she knew said, crazy person. The travails of having a triathlete mother.

"I don't do average, I do awesome."

My children are always incredibly excited about my races. My daughter always insists I enjoy the race while my son wishes for me to "come first". My daughter is on her school swim team, and my son is a natural athlete. I do feel truly blessed that my family understands and wholeheartedly supports my passion for endurance sports.

COVID-19 has brought a lot of things to a standstill, but I took this period as a challenge and worked on my strength training and bike performance. The rewarding part is to see the results. Endurance training is my balancing factor, and it is an essential component of my daily routine. Those who endure, conquer. My Motto.

Never Give Up

All forms of endurance sport need discipline, hard work, integrity and tenacity. To perform and excel, one needs to put heart and soul into it. And above all, you need to enjoy the process. That's my motto. I do believe that this year that shook the world in a not so pleasant manner has not been a waste. It has taught us to love each day, be kind to everyone around us, be mindful of little things and keep looking ahead.

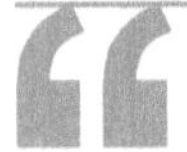

"You're a fighter. Look at everything you've overcome. Don't give up now."

Olivia Benson

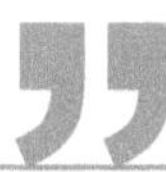

Age or body type should not have anything to do with the confidence you hold. Cross each bridge, each hurdle and each achievement with grace and dignity. Give it's due but move on.

Each one of us faces challenges and personal hardships; there will be days when that pillow seems like the best companion ever. But only when one faces those demons head-on with courage and conviction, can one overcome the odds.

"Wake up with determination. Go to bed with satisfaction."

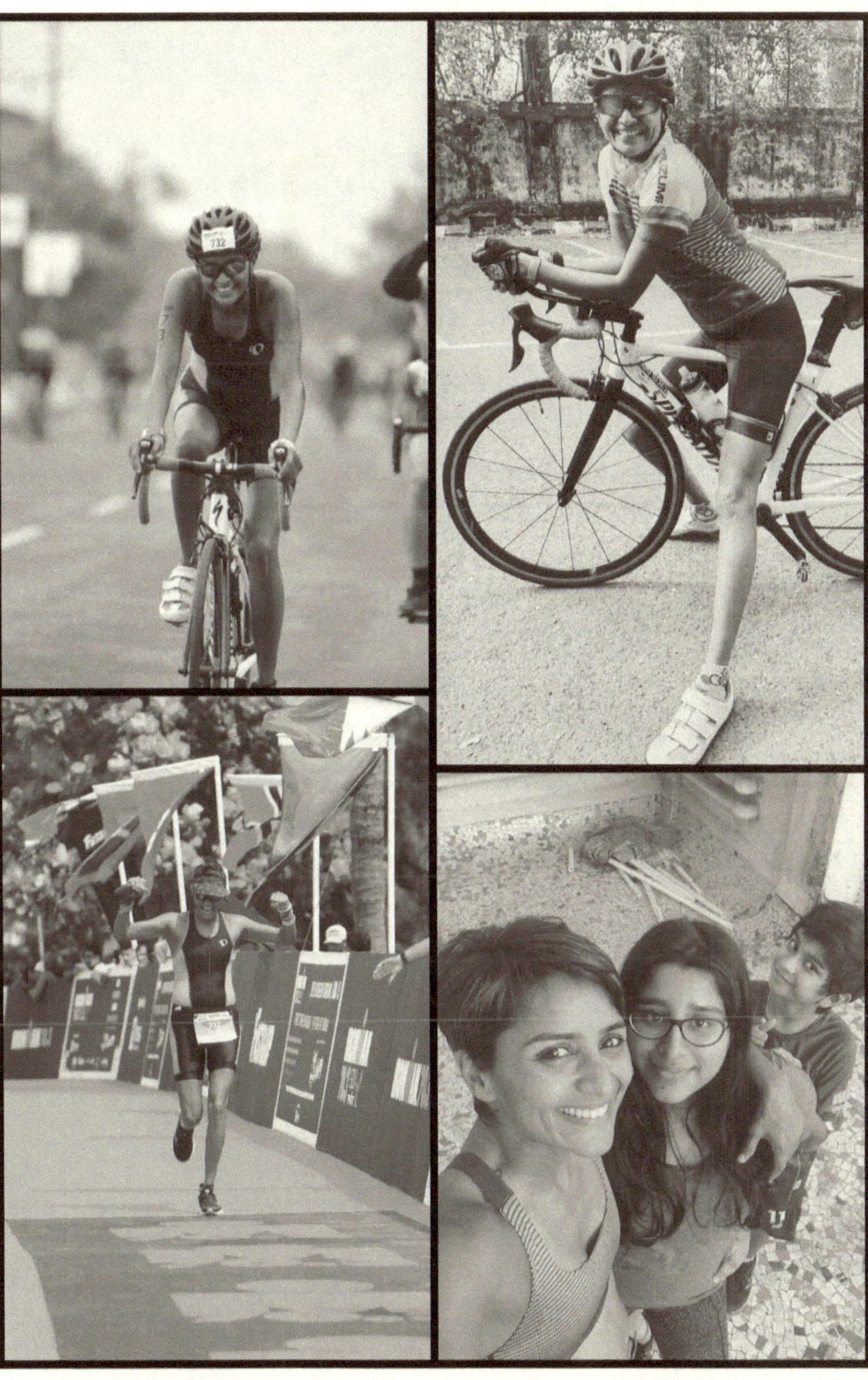

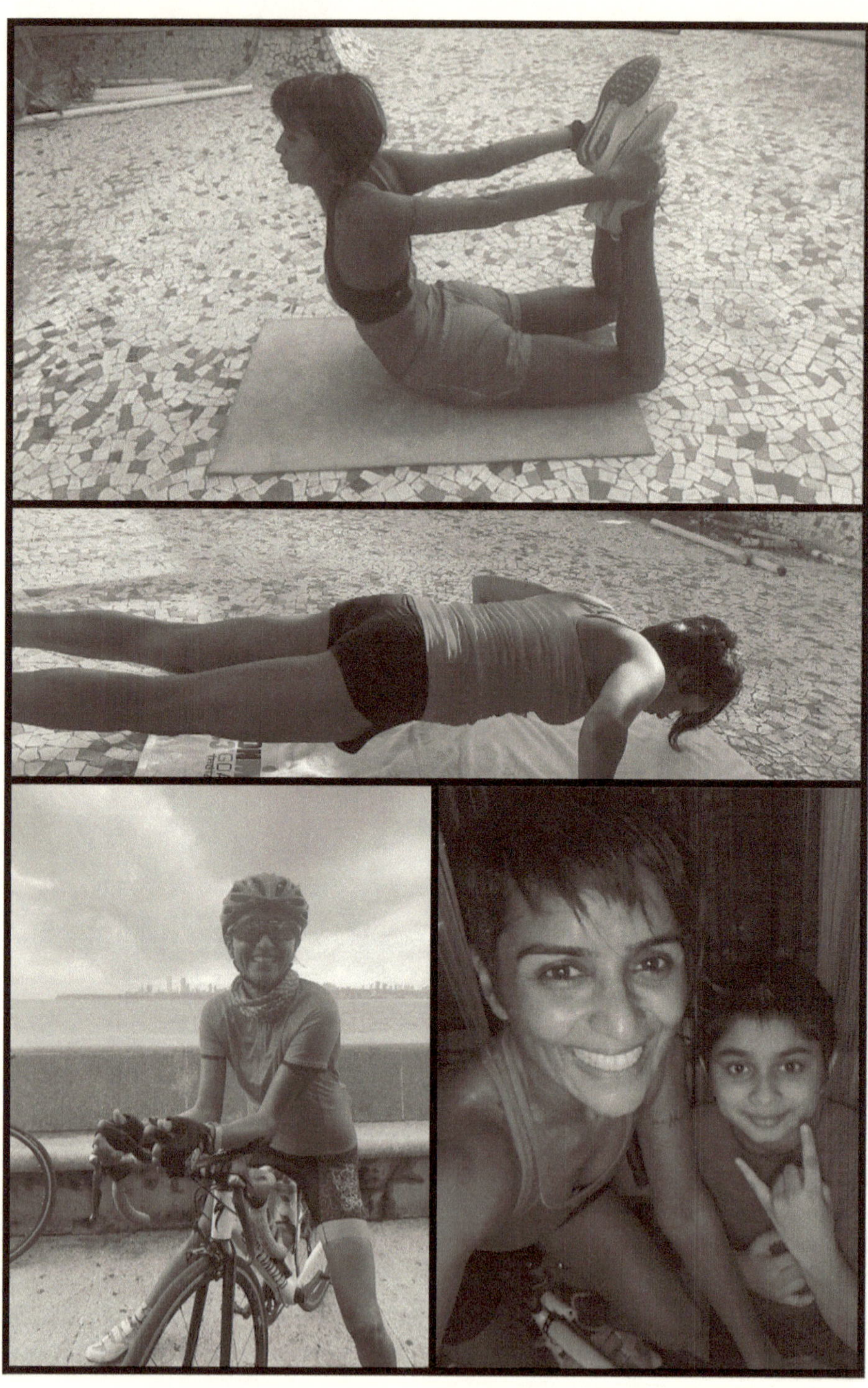

If You Never Give Up 06

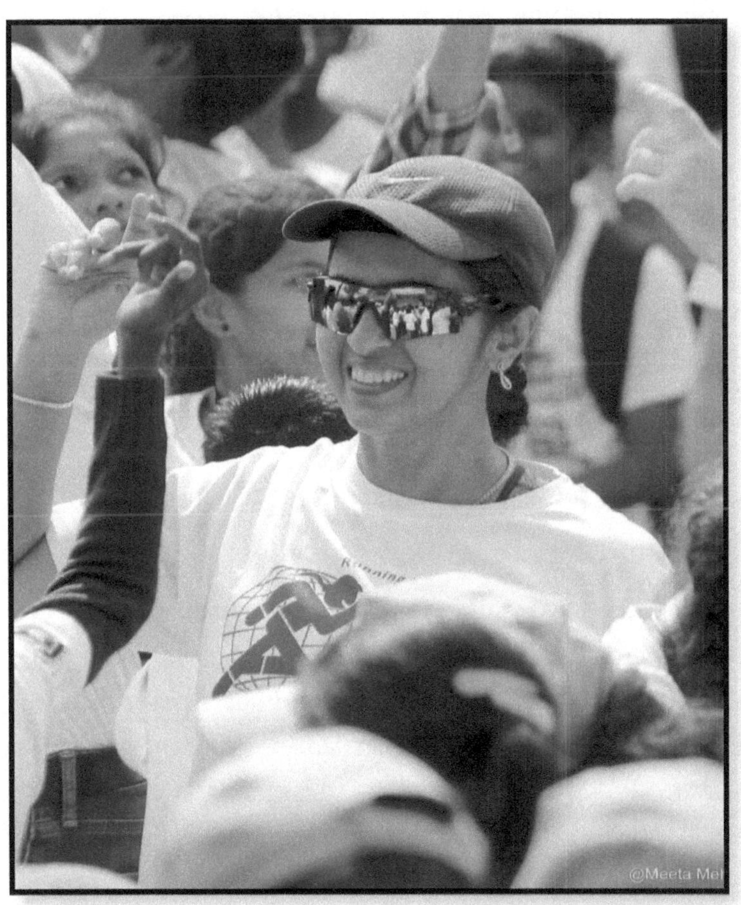

A government official, single mother, persistent failure in all the races, never-ever give up attitude, a robust and daring mother, slow in races but fastest when it comes to catching a local train here is 53-year-old Sree from Mumbai.

The Rough Girl

I was a super naughty girl right from childhood. My parents attended to my complaints more than PTMs. Playing outdoors, bruised knees and bandaged limbs were a regular affair. When I was in grade 8, I fainted while playing in the school. I was rushed to the hospital and was diagnosed with meningitis. I was in a coma for two days. I had many visitors in the hospital, making me feel like a celebrity. It was amusing to know that the visitors were keener to see how a hyper girl can manage to stay in bed for such a long time. The doctors extracted water from my spine and shifted me out of the ICU. They said my recovery was nothing less than a miracle. I was in the hospital for a month.

The doctors informed my parents about the side effects of steroids that I was supposed to take for a year. As expected, I piled on a tremendous amount of weight. I gradually started going for walks and then enrolled myself in taekwondo classes. In a batch of 100, I was the only girl. These classes gave me a lot of confidence and helped me grow in my teens.

I played all sports when I was young – kabaddi, basketball, shot-put, and trekking, among others. My friends called me a "rough girl." I completed my formal education, cleared the SSE exam and got a position in the government postal department. I got married in 1994 and shifted to Kandivali.

When my daughter was a year and a half old, I enrolled myself in a nearby gym. I also joined aerobics and kickboxing. I am an over-enthusiastic individual. I get excited about everything. It was a tedious task to carry on with all the activities along with house chores, taking care of my daughter and work, but I enjoyed everything.

In 2003, a friend took me to the Standard Chartered Mumbai Marathon (SCMM) Dream Run. The electrifying environment made me want to participate again, in 2004.

In 2005 I participated in the half marathon and finished in three hours and 40 minutes. I was shamelessly happy. I continued participating in the SCMM half marathon until 2009.

Then Came the Dark Phase

I was happily enjoying all my activities, work and motherhood. Life had lots to offer, and I was brimming with excitement. Things turned the other way round in 2009 when the word cancer engulfed us. My husband was detected with stage three cancer. Hospital visits, high medical bills and innumerable prescriptions took over my aerobics, dance and kickboxing classes.

His health was deteriorating faster than expected due to diabetes. The doctors asked me to rush him to Cochin to see a specialist. During this process, I fractured my foot, and due to negligence, the recovery period lasted for almost three months. The oncologist in Cochin gave us six months, and I got my husband back to Mumbai.

I had to move around hospitals a lot as my husband wasn't cooperating with the treatment. Gradually his kidneys failed, and after three days of extensive treatment, he finally succumbed to his illness in December 2010. All of a sudden, it was quiet time. All the running around and chaos was over.

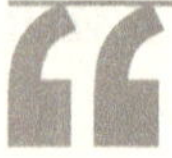

At times silence is also deafening.

I took a while to compose myself and look ahead in life. I had a daughter to raise, and I had no option but to tell myself, "Get up Sree, get going." I resumed work in February 2011.

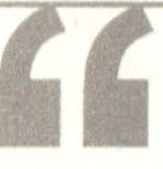

A single sunbeam is enough to drive away many shadows. My daughter was my sunbeam.

Sunny Days Are Here Again

I focused on bringing my life back on track, both physically and mentally. All types of activities had taken a back seat, until 2014, when I came across a training program for runners at the Borivali National Park, on Facebook. The outdoor lover in me and the enthu-cutlet syndrome didn't miss any detail, and I joined the group. I was starting afresh now and was determined to take life my way. I started running regularly. The running location was close to my house hence it was easy to manage 4 am runs, come back home, prepare tiffin, finish household chores and rush to catch the 8 am local to be in the office at 9.30 am. I was gaining back my lost energy. I was happy.

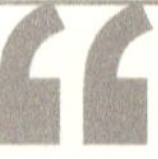

Do what you can, with what you have, where you are.

Theodore Roosevelt

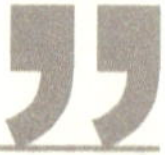

Finished, But Incomplete

Seeing my excitement levels for everything, someone in my running group told me about Triathlons. My only and the biggest worry was – I didn't know how to cycle. Clueless about the sport and out of sheer excitement, I started to learn to cycle in October 2014. I had many falls, and my butt was always sore. I wondered how others happily smile and pose for post-ride pics. Google came to my rescue, and I discovered padded cycling shorts. Rides were not so painful after that. I was not even aware of swimming goggles and would end the session with red and itchy eyes. One of the kids in the pool suggested I wear swimming goggles, and I thank that kid to date.

Here are my finished-yet-incomplete-races.

Goa Triathlon, March 2016

Before the race, I participated in Wada Duathlon to check on my cycling capabilities. The race began with a run of 5 km. After that, I got on my bike to ride 40 km. I barely managed to ride through the off-road track. The villagers took pity on me and asked me to stop if I was unable to cope. I had to finish what I started and did reach the finish line in five and a half hours.

Next was Goa Tri. I packed my bag, laced up my enthusiasm, built up all the courage and traveled to Goa. On the race day, I started the swim peacefully but panicked after 100 meters when I couldn't spot any kayak. But within no time a kayak was near me, he asked me if I wanted to quit, and the reply was a definite no. I told him to be around and finished the 1500 meters. Biking freaks me out, but I mustered all the courage and got on to the bike. After a few loops, a car zoom passed by me, and I slipped on the loose gravel. My front tooth broke, my knee bruised and my face had scratches all over. I wasted 40 minutes contemplating whether I should continue or not.

Then I thought about my sore bums, winter morning swimming sessions, 4 am runs, and with a deep breath, I got up, rubbed my bruises gently, got on to the bike and continued on the course. My bruised knee had swollen severely by now, and I barely managed to finish the run course. Again, I was the last one to reach the finish line. I met my friend Sanjay, and with swollen lips, I managed a small grin showing my broken front tooth.

Chennai Tri, July 2016

I could manage this race in time without any fall.

Pune Tri, November 2016

I went for this race with the confidence and glory of finishing the previous race in time, totally oblivious of the bike route.

I was taken by surprise as the entire biking route was through the ghats. It was a pain-stricken ride, and I finished the race in seven hours when the Half Ironman participants were finishing their race.

After the DNF and abysmal performance in all the races, I was not disappointed; it got me thinking, where did I go wrong? Then I got to know about coaches who guide and train for triathlon participants. I started thinking, which sport was I weakest at, and it took me no time to realize that I wasn't good at any.

Shankar Thapa, a swim coach, came to my rescue. I joined his classes to learn freestyle swimming, as I had only swum breaststroke in all my earlier races. I enrolled in online training plans with Yoksa. I couldn't do justice to my training plans because my workplace shifted, and I spent a lot of time traveling.

Kolhapur Tri, November 2018, 70.3

I was well prepared for this race and was quite hopeful to finish it in time. After a successful swim, I climbed on my bike. After a while, I had difficulty riding. I then realized that the bike tyres were fixed inside out, and I didn't even check while I was assembling my bike. DNF (Did Not Finish), again.

Goa Tri, October 2019, 70.3

Due to massive undercurrents, I drifted while swimming and the kayak informed me that I was going the wrong way. Although I finished the swim, I couldn't make it within the cut-off time, so I aborted the race and went ahead to cheer my fellow mates. DNF (Did Not Finish), again.

Kolhapur Tri, November 2019

First race when everything went fine, and I managed to touch the finish line in five hours and thirty minutes!

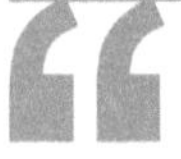

Failure is so important. We speak about success all the time. It is the ability to resist failure or use failure that often leads to greater success. I've met people who don't want to try for fear of failing.

J.K. Rowling

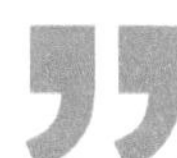

I Was Determined

The days were not easy. Raising my daughter with the compassion of a mother and responsible shoulders of a father was not easy. Being whacked on the bums during early morning runs, dealing with rowdy boys teasing my daughter or rushing from one local to another and then hushing back home from work, I have dealt with all.

Fear is a distant emotion for me. I do not fear the unknown for I have seen and experienced the worst phase in my life. I have also battled domestic violence to a more considerable extent. I also have an accurate observation that I am genetically slow when it comes to races, but no one can beat me when I chase a local train.

My daughter will get married soon, and I'll be on my own. The thought of loneliness doesn't bother me as I am ferociously independent. My daughter and I are best friends and best friends never part.

I had my share of accused and blame games, but I used my two ears wisely. After my husband's demise, people were sure that I would sell my flat and move in with my parents, but I stayed on my own.

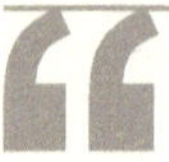

The more you listen, the more you give yourself room for doubt.

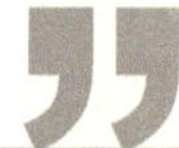

"She is a widow, yet she goes to the gym?"

"She has started working as well!"

"How will she live her entire life without a partner?"

"Can she be a father to her daughter?"

And much more. Ignorance is bliss. I take each day as it comes. I fill each moment with new possibilities, and I aim to live life king size.

If I Can

If I can stand up for myself, learn to fall and cycle at the age of 46; when I can face all my DNFs with triumph. If I can listen and yet not get affected by whatever society says or expects from me, anyone can muster the courage and live a life filled with gratitude and self-respect. One day

I'll finish Ironman 70.3 within time and will grin ear to ear without a broken tooth.

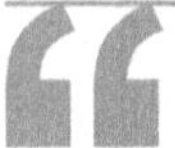

"The woman you're becoming will cost you people, relationships, spaces and material things. Choose her over everything."

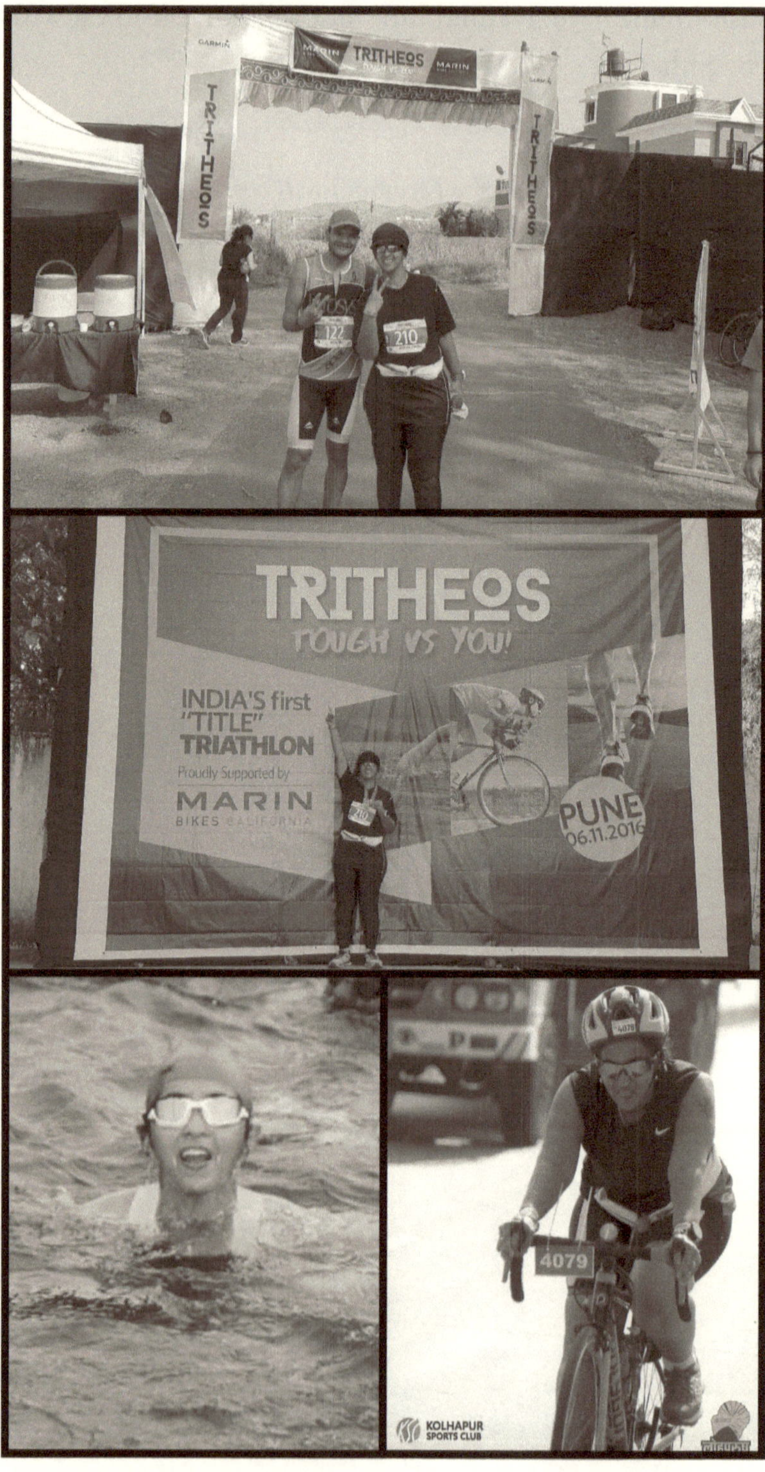
TRITHEOS
TOUGH VS YOU!
INDIA'S first
"TITLE"
TRIATHLON
Proudly Supported by
MARIN
BIKES CALIFORNIA
PUNE
06.11.2016
KOLHAPUR
SPORTS CLUB

No Joy in the Easy; No Fear of the Tough

07

If I Can, Then Anyone Can Become An Ironman

Charanya Ravikumar, Texas

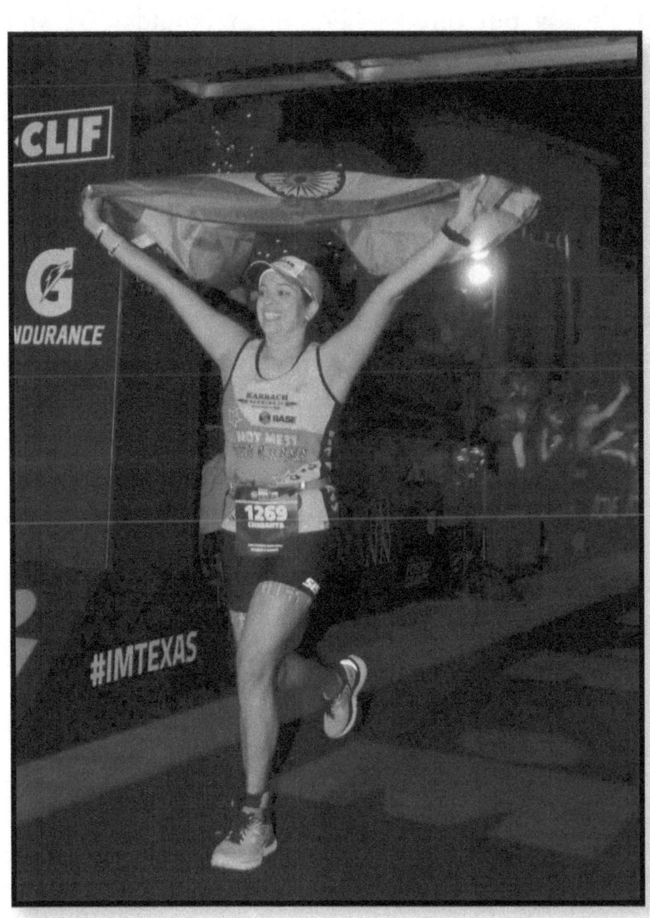

Beyond barriers and hindrances, she found her own inspiration and went behind it. She touched finish lines she had never even dreamed of – a computer engineer, a social sector professional, an accidental triathlete, a full ironman finisher, one of the few Indian women to finish 140.6, a mother of two and the wife of an aspiring Ironman, an Indian by heart and birth, she's Charanya Ravikumar.

I was born in India but moved to Singapore soon after, where I completed schooling and moved to the U.S. for higher education in 2001. I was the last bencher when it came to participating in any sports activity. I was more into debates and drama than anything sporty.

I got hooked to the American lifestyle pretty quickly and by the time I realized it, I had already put on the "Freshman Pounds 15" and more! Staying healthy was not a priority for me. After completing my professional education, I started working with Dell. The work environment made me conscious of my weight. I was looking for ways to shed the extra pounds but couldn't find one.

I finally came across Asha for Education, a non-profit organization that trained aspiring runners for marathons to raise funds for kids back in India through its program, Strides of Hope. I was always keen to contribute and create awareness about issues impacting kids, and what better way to do that than running!

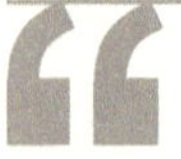

"The marathon is not really about the marathon; it's about the shared struggle. And it's not only the marathon but the training."

Bill Buffum

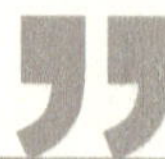

I trained hard to reach my first half-marathon finish line in 2007, and thoroughly enjoyed the experience. The sense of community and the finisher's high made me immediately sign up for my first full marathon – the Marine Corps Marathon in Washington DC.

A New Love Was Blooming

I participated in the Marine Corps Marathon in 2007 and it was a scintillating experience. The course runs along many of the iconic national monuments of Washington D.C. The event focuses on strengthening community spirit, promoting good health and showcasing the organizational skills of the United States Marines. For these reasons, it has rightly earned its nickname as "The People's Marathon". There were runners from Asha for Education from across the country, and it was a great feeling to run together.

In due course, I ran seven marathons, never repeating a course and using the run as a great way to explore a new city and collect fancy medals as well. Around the same time, a friend who had signed up for a Sprint Triathlon relay was looking for a swimmer. I was supposed to swim 800 meters, and I readily agreed. Swimming was a part of my school curriculum, so it was not a big deal for me. Well, not until I reached the venue and got to know that the swim was in a lake and not in a pool!

Once I got into the water though, my nervousness vanished and it ended up being a beautiful experience. I even bumped into a friendly turtle! While I waited for the race to get over, I got to experience the energy, the adrenaline rush, and the camaraderie – it was palpable. I was as excited as a child going to Disneyland for the first time. I started participating in sprint distance triathlons and did two to three races a year. I had found my new love!

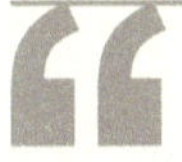

"There is no one giant step that does it. It's a lot of little steps".

Difficult Road, Fulfilling Destination

I was working at Dell, but the work didn't excite me, so as soon as I could, I left my job and started volunteering for various causes. I also ended up pregnant at this time and before I knew it, my baby boy was six months old, and I was wholly engrossed in mom duties as well as dealing with mild postpartum blues. I had made my own decision to leave work, take care of my baby and volunteer, but I was not happy. I felt like I was not doing anything meaningful and my postpartum body brought me back to my post-college days. With no childcare support, it was tricky to figure out how to start incorporating a workout routine.

"Wise people say, you will find a way if you put your heart to it."

I came across a club called Stroller Strides in the vicinity where the workouts took place around the baby's stroller. I enjoyed those sessions, and it was a stepping stone towards my fitness journey. Meanwhile, I also started going for spin classes and started getting back into form, slowly and steadily.

In Jan 2014, I learned about Ironman Galveston 70.3 coming up in April 2014, and enthusiastically signed up for it. I trained on my own as I wasn't aware of proper training plans or other nuances. Managing training between nursing and tending to the baby and household was a challenging task, but I managed to finish in eight hours and twenty-nine minutes, just a minute below the cutoff! I decided I would train better and come back and do the same race next year, but I got pregnant instead, and only managed to go back three years later in 2017.

I had a baby girl now and my older toddler boy to manage along with my training, and a full-time job. It was a herculean task to train while managing full-time work, taking care of the kiddos, and trying to have a semblance of a social life!

It was my first experience training with a coach and a structured training plan. I had a lot of inhibitions with interacting and communicating with my coach. I felt guilty if I missed a workout. I also hesitated to talk about issues like cramps and periods (not being able to talk openly about periods is not an issue in India alone but all over the globe).

I attempted the race again and improved by only 45 minutes. I had hoped to do a lot better! But I had a fire in my belly. I wanted to improve. I wanted to emerge stronger. I wanted to be more than just a wife or mom or employee. I decided to push myself toward the ultimate triathlete goal, I signed up for full Ironman.

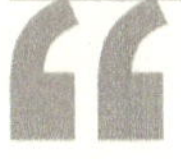

"Don't think about the start of the race, think about the ending."

Usain Bolt

"Quitters don't tri. Triathletes don't quit — The full Ironman."

I firmly believe in this quote

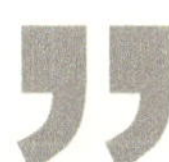

I knew that I wasn't the strongest or fastest athlete, but I also knew that I was not a quitter. A full Ironman requires total dedication and sincere hard work. I was ready to give it my all.

I needed guidance and a structured approach and a coach I was completely comfortable with. My friend Tim from my local Tri club was aspiring to be a coach, and I readily agreed to be his guinea pig. Tim's plans were completely structured toward accommodating my crazy schedule, but at the same time planned well to move me from strength to strength toward my goal. I was completely comfortable discussing my shortcomings, and scope for improvement. I accomplished my training goals one week at a time.

In 2018, with six months of dedicated training, I attempted my first full Ironman, Ironman Texas and finished in 15:56:58. Neither the training nor the race was easy. Well, if it was easy, then why would I have attempted it?

> *"When you run the marathon, you run against the distance, not against the other runners and not against the time."*
>
> **Haile Gebrselassie**

On the race day, after the cheering and hugs from fellow participants and family members, I headed for the swim course. As I started my swim, the next wave entered the water, and I was surrounded by a swarm of swimmers. One swimmer almost pulled out my timing chip, and I had to get into the treading water position to fix it, and in the process gulped a lot of the nasty water. I was conscious all through the swim course about my loose timing chip and stopped many times to check on it. Almost midway, I could feel my stomach churning, but there was no way I was stopping. I finished the swim in 1:37:04.

The bike course started fine, and I was on target as planned. My stomach was still churning, but nothing serious. 20 minutes in, I took a sip of my electrolyte drink and immediately threw up. My stomach wasn't accepting anything, and I kept throwing up. When I reached mile 62, I tried to have a jam and cheese sandwich and kept praying that I shouldn't throw up anymore. Miraculously I didn't. It was a big relief. I was slowly regaining strength. I also found a photo of my kids my husband Vish had packed for me with the sandwich, and it surged me with instant energy. I finished the bike course in 8hr: 07min: 19sec, an hour more than the plan.

The three-loop run course though was an absolute delight. I loved the crowd support, constant cheering, nutrition stations with fresh watermelon, and the overall positive energy. I loved seeing and high-fiving my kids, husband, parents, coach, teammates, colleagues and friends who had all shown up at the race. I felt like a rockstar.

I wasn't tired and was enjoying every moment of the last lap. I was gliding and could feel the energy flow in me. As I approached the finish line, I saw Coach Tim and handed over my water belt to him, and he passed me the Indian flag. I crossed the finish line holding the flag up, high and rising. I finished the run in 5hr: 45min: 52sec

During my entire race, I wasn't bothered about my overall finish time. I was careful about meeting the timing cutoffs of course, but I was committed right from the beginning to enjoying my race and giving it my best!

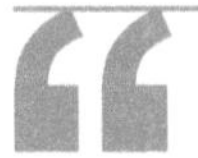

"To be a triathlete means to have the adapted body and mind to endure a challenge that motivates yourself and all who know you."

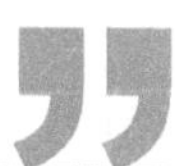

The last 30 seconds were the most incredible moments I had ever experienced in my life, second only to giving birth to my two babies!

Finding Inspiration All Around

Several incidents inspired me to take up this sport. My memories go back to my first relay sprint triathlon where I was awestruck by the energetic environment. Volunteering once at Ironman Texas made me see the grit and determination of athletes. My husband Vishwas and I volunteered at one of the last water stops and witnessed athletes of all ages, sizes and shapes making it to the finish line.

In a recent half-marathon, I saw a group of women who were over 60 years old, holding hands and crossing the finish line. Their energy and joy were infectious and reminded me why I indulge in these sports. Training for a race and crossing the finish line with your buddies is just an exhilarating feeling – I will take this over partying any day!

With so much inspiration around us, it is easy to tap into your potential and take that first step, be it towards going to the gym, signing up for a 5K, or even showing up at a Stroller Strides workout with your baby. Once you motivate yourself to take that initial step, things will start to shape up and fall into place.

For any activity that involves a woman stepping out of the house, it is infinitely easier when there is complete buy-in from the family. There's no concept of house-help abroad. Everything has to be done on our own. Although daycare facilities and childcare at gyms are more readily available here than in India, the support and understanding from the family is still a must.

I have been asked many times about the need to indulge in triathlons with a small baby or two small children, questioned about leaving my children alone with my husband while training etc., but thankfully never from my own family. Vish has always been 150% on board with my goals from day one. He understood my passion and my desire to do something for myself – in this case, to participate in endurance sports. He is a born athlete and an avid runner. He started to learn to swim after we met, motivated to do triathlons as well. He would have completed his first Ironman this year if not for COVID-19. We have run during our travels, including doing a half-marathon during our honeymoon!

Our kids are used to seeing one parent missing on weekend mornings and question us if we choose to sleep in. We love setting an example for our kids, and they are excited to do their first kids' triathlons down the road as well.

Onward and Upward

I have done the distances I've wanted to do, but I would love to continue becoming a stronger athlete. I would love to participate in races all over the world, including India! I also want to see more South Asian women participating in endurance sports. It puzzles me why few women who look like me at the races despite living in a country that has top-notch facilities for athletes – and have found that a lot of the barriers that women in India face are present across the diaspora as well.

Down the line, when I can devote the time and effort, I would love to work with young girls and women and encourage them to take up endurance sports and help them realize what they can all be capable of! Women can and should be able to do anything they decide to do!

A Strong Woman Raises a Strong Family

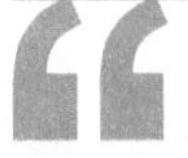

"You don't have to be so tough that it doesn't hurt; you just have to be tough enough not to quit."

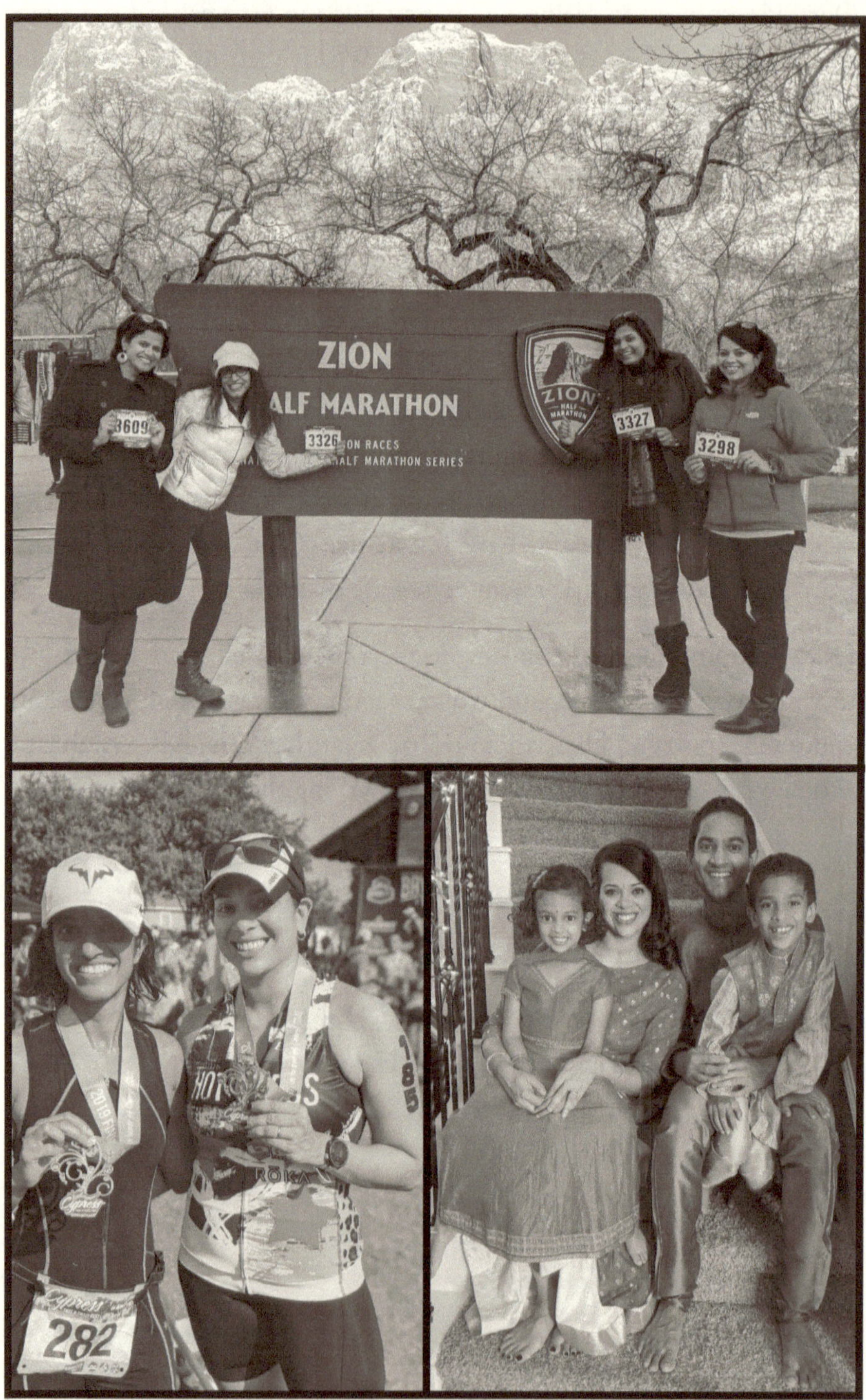
ZION
ALF MARATHON
ON RACES
HALF MARATHON SERIES
ZION
HALF
MARATHON
3609
3326
3327
3298
282

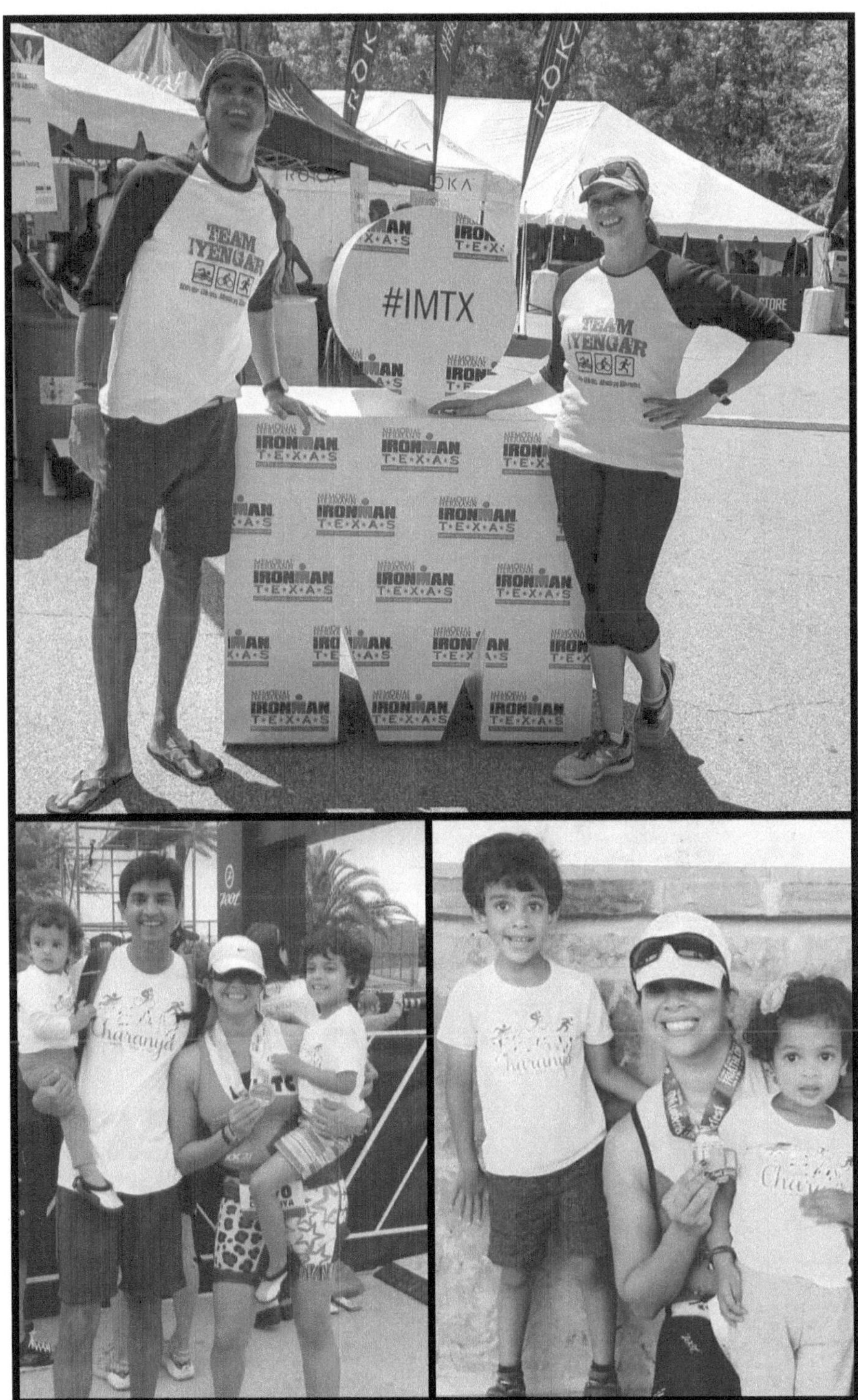
TEAM IYENGAR
#IMTX
TEAM IYENGAR
IRONMAN
T·E·X·A·S

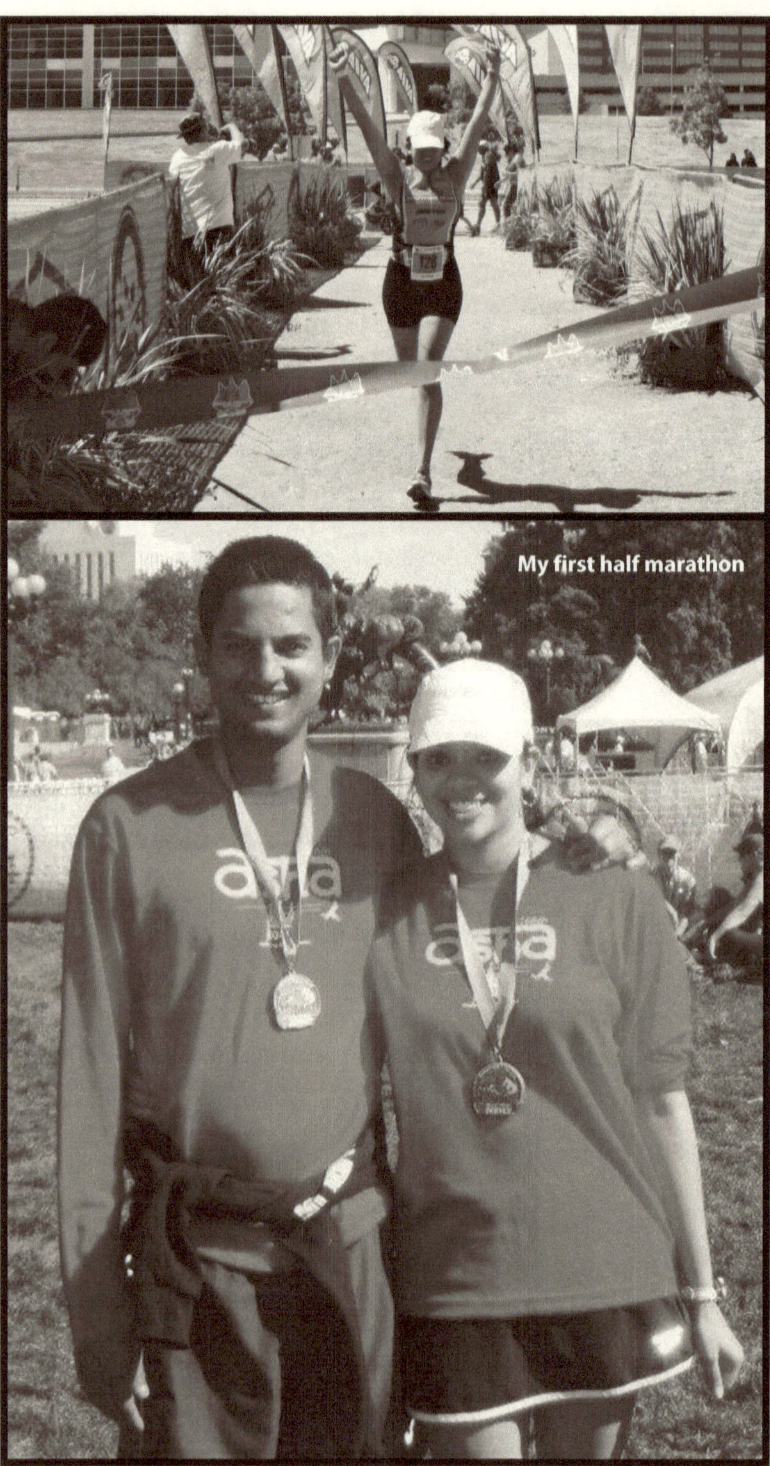
My first half marathon

She Runs with Her Heart

Curvy and Cheeky, Attitude Knows No Boundaries

Ami Paneri

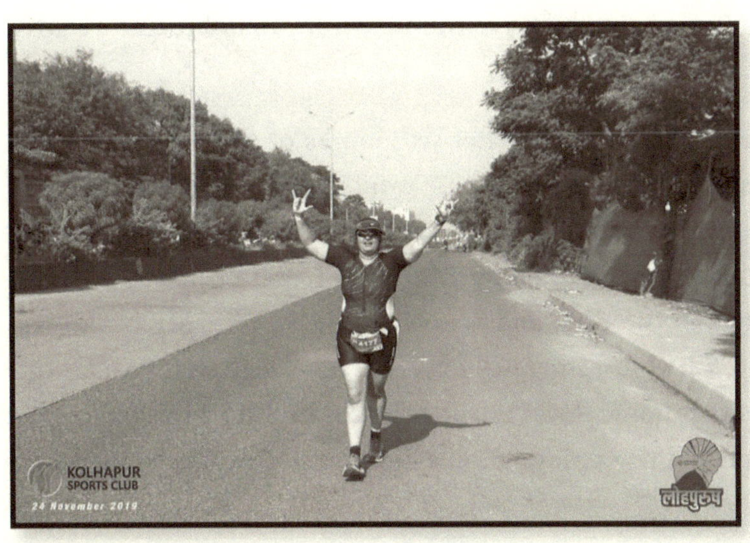

Bodyweight was the biggest demon in her life – physically, mentally and emotionally. But that didn't pull her down. She chose to run it out. Now she runs free with all her heart and grit. An IT professional, progressive runner, determined triathlete, self-motivator, nothing weighs her down – a total novice in the athletic world, cycling lover, mother of two – Ami Paneri from Mumbai loves to run marathons and triathlons.

Motherhood and the Aftermath

I was the eldest of three siblings, always an obedient and studious girl. I loved playing with electronic items more than dolls, thanks to my dad. He worked in ISRO, and gadgets were a significant part of discussions in the house. I was an outdoor child. Playing in the wild, running on trails, and burning the skin under the sun were my favorite things.

I learned cycling on hired Tobo bikes and got my first personal cycle when I was in grade 6. It was a prized possession. Since then, the cycle was my mode of transport to school and then to college as well. I completed my MSc, M. Phil, and secured a gold medal in computer science. In 2007, I got married and shifted to Mumbai from Gandhinagar. I started working as an ERP professional.

In 2008 I had my first child. After six months of maternity leave, due to several reasons, I could not resume work. I was loaded with heaps of responsibilities of a young child, a mother-in-law, and myself. I faced the most challenging time between 2009–11, the postpartum phase. I was irritable all the time and was piling on weight. My health was deteriorating. I had lost interest in everything. There were regular tiffs and arguments at home. I was missing myself. In 2011 I had my second child. I weighed a whopping 90 plus kgs now. I gradually started with regular gym and weight training. I loved that one hour in the morning, all to myself.

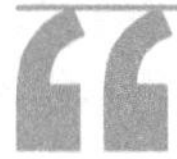

> *Motherhood is joyous, but it can also be overwhelming. Everyone congratulates you on having a baby, but no one warns about the aftermath, mainly postpartum depression.*

Gaining Back My Confidence

It's said that I speak "heavy" words, but now I was proving it correct. I was so heavy that I became self-conscious all the time. I would avoid going to public places, meeting people, and would avoid the gym if it was crowded. I would avoid arms workouts at the gym as the bulge embarrassed me.

In 2011, my husband participated in the Standard Chartered Mumbai Marathon (SCMM) Dream Run, and I went along. The electrifying environment zapped me. I wanted to be there – running. I wanted that zeal and energy – and I had none. The best thing that happened during this time was, I got back to work. It was a welcoming change. I was happy to move out and sort my routine.

In 2013, I participated in the SCMM half marathon and somehow managed to drag myself and reach the finish line in 3.37 hours. I realized what it takes to run and finish. I had no idea about training, so I started running independently. I managed between kids, work, and home. In 2015 I participated in the SCMM half marathon and finished in an abysmal timing of 3.58 hours. I hadn't progressed; I had digressed. I was missing out on something, but couldn't figure out what.

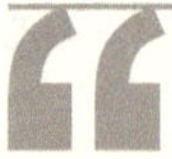

"You're so much more than the numbers on your plus size lingerie"

In 2016, I joined Pinkathon. I was incredibly body-conscious and would run before the sunshine to hide from the eyes watching an overweight female trying to run. Pinkathon helped me realize that many like are struggling with body shaming and the social stigma attached to it. I had lots of co-sisters sailing in the same boat. I gradually gained confidence and started running in a group.

In 2016, a friend organized Wada Duathlon and asked me to participate. I was thrilled. I got my cycle, and my long-lost love was back in full form. Cycling was my childhood love, and once I am on my bike, I am the happiest person around. I gradually started coming back to my happy and confident form.

In 2017 I participated In Wada Duathlon yet again and stood first. In the same year, I did my first 80 km ride to Kharghar with the Malad cycling club. Ah! I was flying.

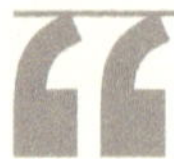

"When the spirits are low, when the day appears dark, when work becomes monotonous, when hope hardly seems worth having, just mount a bicycle and go out for a spin down the road, without thought on anything but the ride you are taking."

Sir Arthur Conan Doyle (1859 – 1930), author of Sherlock Holmes

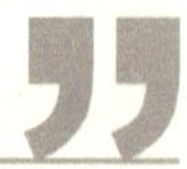

The Ladakh Marathon

In 2018 My husband registered for the Ladakh marathon and I wanted to participate as well. After booking the flight tickets with an overdose of excitement, the reality came crashing on me. I didn't fit the eligibility criterion. I did not have a required timing certificate. Viv came to my rescue. What would I ever do without his meticulous training plans? When I shared my desire to participate in the marathon, he gladly welcomed my thought and encouraged me to train hard. I participated in several 10 K runs.

I was chasing races and timing. I was desperate. And finally, from 1.40hrs, I managed 1.18hrs for a 10K run. What a delight! I had the timing certificate, and I was going for the Ladakh marathon. I finished the marathon, and it was a great confidence booster for me.

Trying the Tri

Our training group, MMA (Mad Menon Academy), is always buzzing with interesting discussions. During one such discussion, the term 'triathlon' caught my attention. Further, I found out that a triathlon is a combination of three sports – swimming, cycling, and running – one after the other. As I mentioned, heavy is my second name, so I took this "heavy" decision to participate in the Kolhapur triathlon 2018.

The primary issue was – I didn't know how to swim. Swimming, for me, was splashing in the water and nothing more. My husband, Sopan, became my teammate. I would take him to a 25 meters pool and ask him to stand at a distance of 15 meters, enough for me to push myself from one end, float, and then hold me to start the same process all over again until I finish the entire lap. I would also refrain from putting my head down in the water.

Shankar Thapa came as a guiding light. I gradually improved my swimming from 15–100–500–700 to finally 1000 meters. With all the training and hard work, I was still not losing weight.

As William Blake said, *"The true method of knowledge is an experiment."* So, I did all it could take to shed the extra kilos. The catch here was that I was following google knowledge, and in this process, I compromised on my immunity. I had worked hard, but my health was not in good shape. Still, with a firm thought and a belief to reach the finish line, I along with my husband, headed to Kolhapur to participate in our first Triathlon. We both panicked in the open water swim, and it was a DNF.

In February 2019, I participated in my home turf, Gandhinagar Triathlon. It was a pool swim with a uniform depth across the pool. As I jumped in the pool, I panicked again. The lifeguards prompted me to pull me out, but I requested them to give me a few minutes to regain my composure. I was angry with myself. I took a deep breath, asked my mind to shut up, and firmly told myself, "Ami, this can't happen again, just go for it", and I go for it, I did. I swam through the entire distance.

I finished the Olympic Distance in 4 hours and 21 minutes. I had to complete the unfinished battle. In November 2019, I participated in the Kolhapur triathlon, this time for the Olympic distance. I finished it in 4 hours 29 minutes. I shall continue to work hard under my coach's guidance and will try to improve in the upcoming races.

Curves and the Social Stigma

I have faced enough questions about my weight. I have hidden under large clothing, covered my arms and ran alone, so that people won't see me. I hid for a very long time.

"If losing weight was easy, we would all be skinny."

Steven Magee

Participating in the running and triathlon events, with the support and encouragement from the family, fellow runners, and coach, I accepted myself as me. I can now run in broad daylight, wear cycling shorts, and swim in a bikini. I have overcome all body shame, and here I stand beholding my confidence firm in my gait, and yes, I still use "heavy" words!

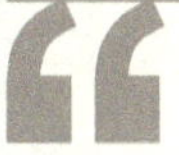

You are beautiful because of the light you carry inside you. You are beautiful because you say you are, and you hold yourself that way.

Mary Lambert

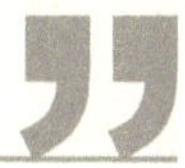

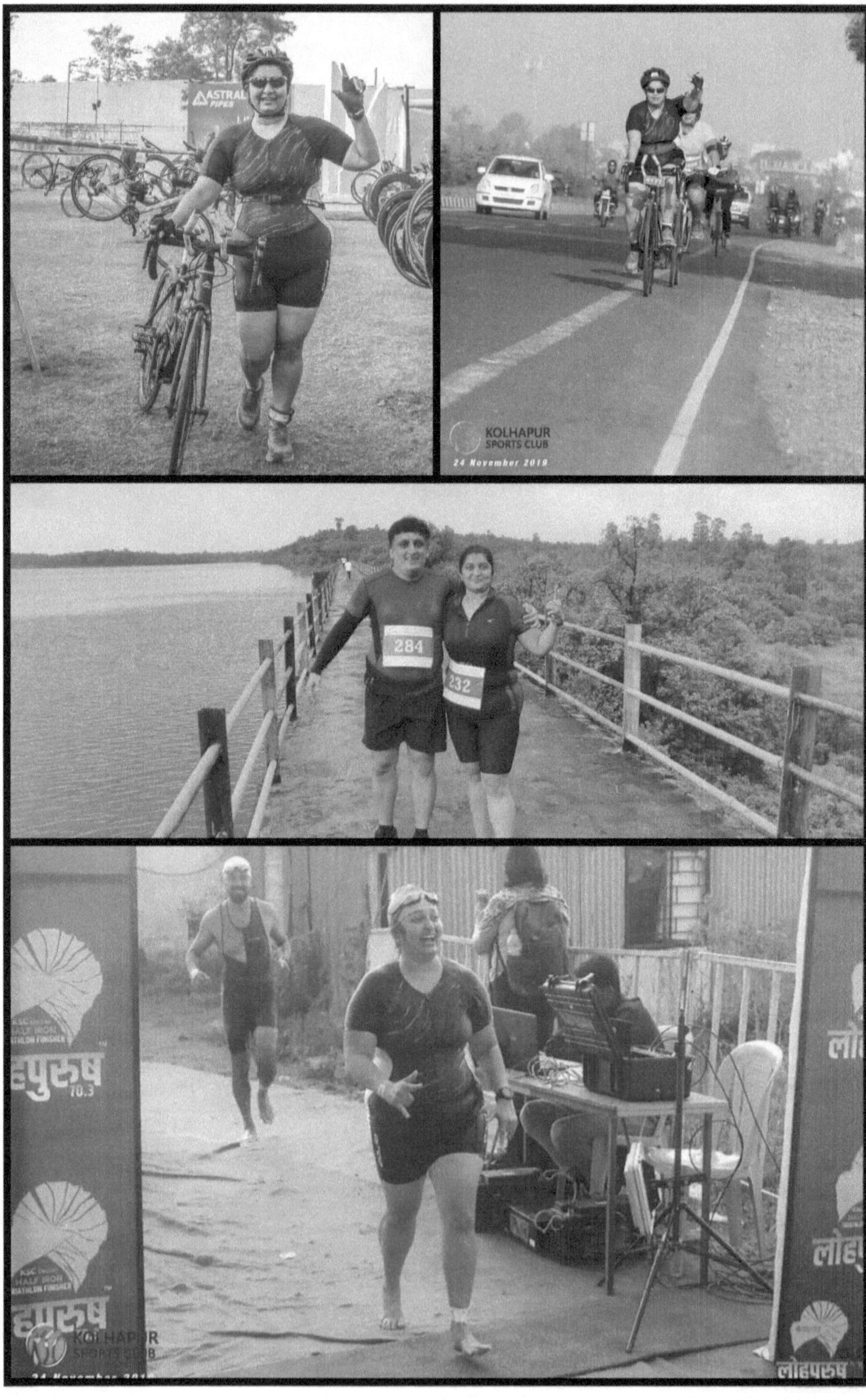

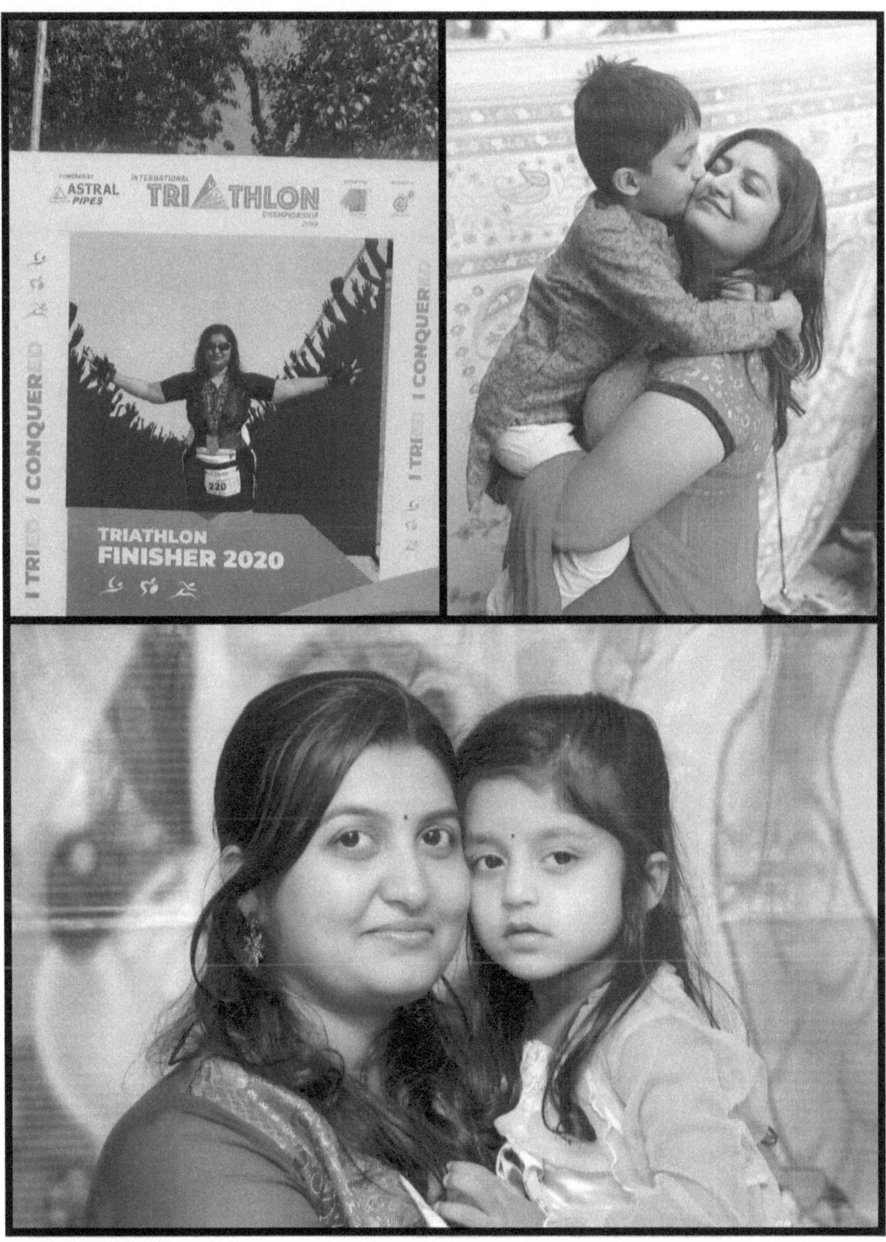

POWERED BY ASTRAL PIPES
INTERNATIONAL
TRIATHLON
CHAMPIONSHIP
I TRIED I CONQUERED
I TRIED I CONQUERED
TRIATHLON
FINISHER 2020
220

Passion Knows No Obstacles | 09

Dabang Maa

Sunita Dhote, Nagpu

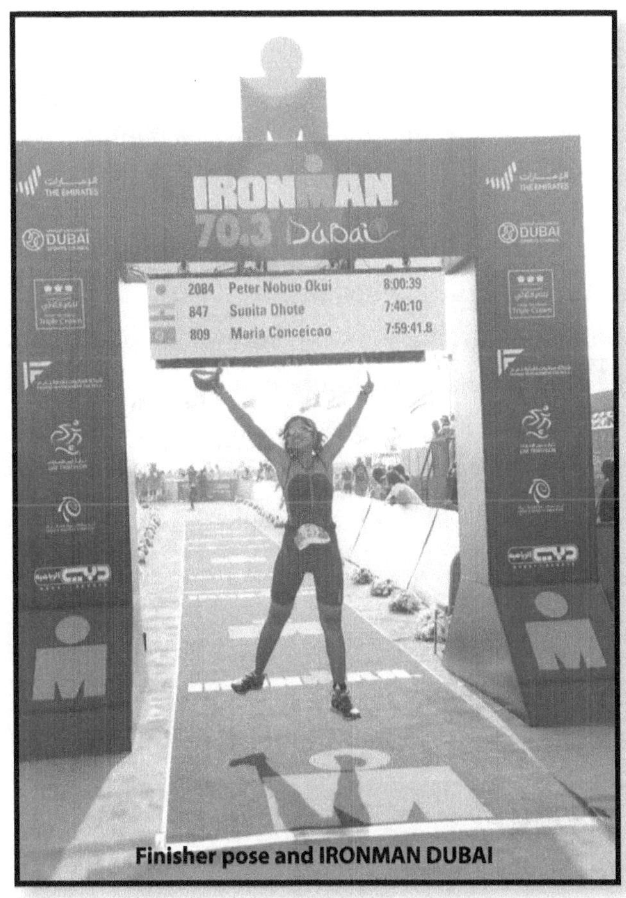

Finisher pose and IRONMAN DUBAI

Mother of two boys, Asia Book of Records holder, represented India in Canada for somersault competition, a college professor; from three failed Ironman attempts to a successful finish, a woman who stood for her passion in a family where her only role was household chores, this is Nagpur-based 48-year-old Sunita Dhote's perspective on life as a winner.

Army Home Childhood

My father was in the Indian Air Force, and I've been brought up all over India. I call myself '*Bharat Ki Beti*' (Daughter of India). My childhood was strict, full of discipline. My father used to wake us up (myself and my younger brother) at 5 am, and we were then supposed to take four rounds of the park in the vicinity. Any mischievous act or cheating would result in additional drills. We learned cycling on hired bikes for a rent of 10 paise per hour. Mistakes would result in tight slaps. I was annoyed at that time, but now I understand the significance of discipline that my father instilled in us.

I was into sports from the beginning. I got selected for the state high jump when papa was posted in Guwahati. I wasn't allowed to participate in nationals because of the fear that high jump would make me taller, and I won't get a desirable match. By the time I reached my tenth grade, sport was just a memory. My entire focus shifted towards studies. I did my B.com, M.com, MBA, and Ph.D. I was an obedient daughter.

Marriage and the Grind

I got married in a business family, and as soon as I entered my in-law's place, all the maids were laid off. I was a full-time maid now. Right from washing clothes, utensils, and cooking, every chore was my responsibility. I have no regret; instead, I am grateful to my mother-in-law for teaching me patience. She cribbed and I listened.

This habit taught me how not to react unnecessarily and carry on with my task. She made me physiologically strong-a much-needed trait for an athlete. It was during my honeymoon to Nepal that I had a glimpse of the golden pagodas. I wanted to run to the top and share the desire with my husband. He gladly agreed, and within no time, I saw myself running on the trail towards the pagoda. The hidden sportsperson in me was still alive. When I reached the top, a stranger shared a message; my husband was waiting for me. He didn't climb.

At this point, I decided, my children will not be the ones waiting down but the ones who would climb the fastest.

I finished my Ph.D. in 2011 and settled for a job. I understood that it was essential to be financially independent. Having traveled all across India with my father, I was a keen traveler but never got an opportunity post-marriage. During one of the exchange programs, I got an opportunity to travel to Seattle and stay at the Microsoft research center. I loved the experience of being on my own and interacting with people across the globe. I was impressed by their discipline, eating habits, and zing for life. I came back with a determination – I have to take charge of my life. I will not fall into this rut.

The Beginning

The group study exchange program to Seattle was a game-changer. Another episode that triggered my thought process was when I was an entrepreneurship faculty, and I talked to students about passion. I read many autobiographies in this process, and each story had one primary learning – follow your passion. It filled me with energy and determination.

After my first son was born, I started to learn swimming. I wasn't allowed to swim in my childhood because if I turn dark, I won't get a suitable match, my parents thought. I used to go to the pool nearby, considering all the eyes watching me or even following. I used to hide my swimming costume in a towel, dry my hair, and dress up "appropriately" for this adventure.

In 2012, I stood first in the 100 meters butterfly championship. I now wanted to learn more. So, I went ahead and learned diving. I was allowed to carry on with whatever I wished to with the condition that children should not be neglected and the house was well attended. So, I used to take my children along with me to the pool. In this process, they also learned swimming (a win-win situation).

Within five to six years, I was a diving champion. Even then, I was struggling at somersault. I pleaded with a child in the pool to teach me. I was 41 years old at that point. That child made me do 100 meters of front and roll and said confidently, "You are ready." I could now do front and reverse somersaults.

I represented India in 2014 in Canada for somersault championships. It was an enthralling moment when I heard my name, Sunita Dhote, India. I was beginning to enjoy my life filled with confidence and joy. To add to my newly discovered joy, I did solo cycling from Nagpur to Pondicherry – a total distance of 1412 km in six days and registered my name in the Asia book of records.

Failure to Finish Line

In 2017 a friend introduced the word Triathlon to me. With an assumption that it's just swimming, cycling, and running, I enrolled for Pune Triathlon, sprint distance. To my dismay, after the swim and the bike, I couldn't manage to run.

Being a total novice, I participated in the race empty stomach. I was unaware of the word nutrition. The same year, I enrolled for the

Hyderabad Triathlon, and it was a DNF. I attempted thrice and failed. Me being me, I don't leave until done.

In 2018, finally, I could finish the race in nine hours and 15 minutes. A friend told me about systematic training, planning, and nutrition. I then took proper coaching and participated in the Dubai Ironman. Ten days before the race, I had two bad falls, and my training came to a standstill. But I am a stubborn soul, and I was determined to fly to Dubai for the race.

I swam for the first time in a wetsuit, and the clear water gave a feeling of *"patal lok"* I clocked my PB in the swim. Cycling was comfortable, and during the run, I followed a strategy to run pole to pole. My Dubai Ironman finish was blissfully satisfying. I became the first woman from the Vidarbha region to have completed the Ironman race.

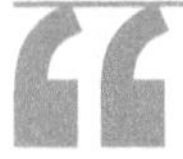

When life gives you restrictions, don't flutter in a cage; instead, look for that one little opportunity to fly out.

When I came back and showed the medal to my family, my husband had a blank expression, and he could only ask me, "Iske liye itni mehnat? (so much of effort just for this medal?)"

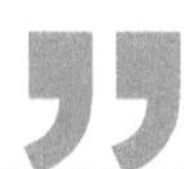

It's sometimes difficult to explain your desires and passion, so it's better to keep the hustle on and move forward. The training was a tricky part. I used to put a cycle in my car, wear cycling gear, and cover it with a salwar suit (formal dress). Once college used to get over, I drove to the highway, parked my car, did a three-hour cycle, and returned home. There were several episodes where I had to manage the timing and surroundings efficiently.

Life's All About Perspectives

When I did my solo cycling, my elder son was in grade 10. I had to listen to a lot of "*gyan*" from everyone about how I was an irresponsible mother who had left her son behind in the crucial year. During a press conference for the Asia book of records, a media person had serious doubts about my grit and daring to do a solo ride. I wanted to ask him," Are you scared of a woman being on her own or are you feeling insecure?"

I didn't allow life to churn me. I did the other way round. I fund my races. I ensured that I brought up my boys with discipline and integrity. Work colleagues who once questioned my caliber now have the utmost respect for me. My son does 200 crunches, and we are quite competitive about it (in all humor). He also cooks a fantastic meal.

My nickname is Sona (gold), and one property of gold is that it glitters the most when it is rubbed hard and rough.

It is my time to glow, and I'll ensure that I shine the brightest.

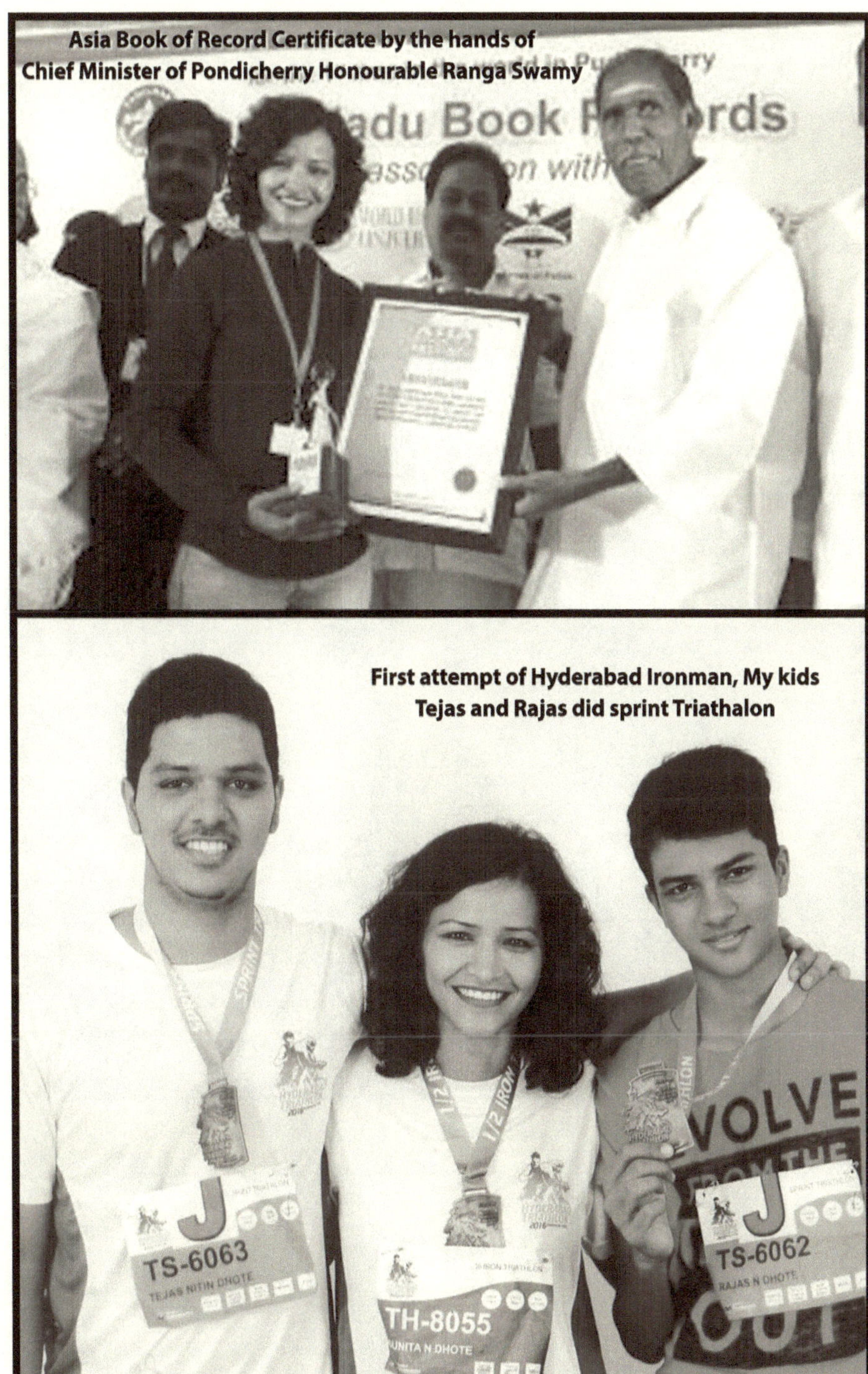
Asia Book of Record Certificate by the hands of
Chief Minister of Pondicherry Honourable Ranga Swamy

First attempt of Hyderabad Ironman, My kids
Tejas and Rajas did sprint Triathalon

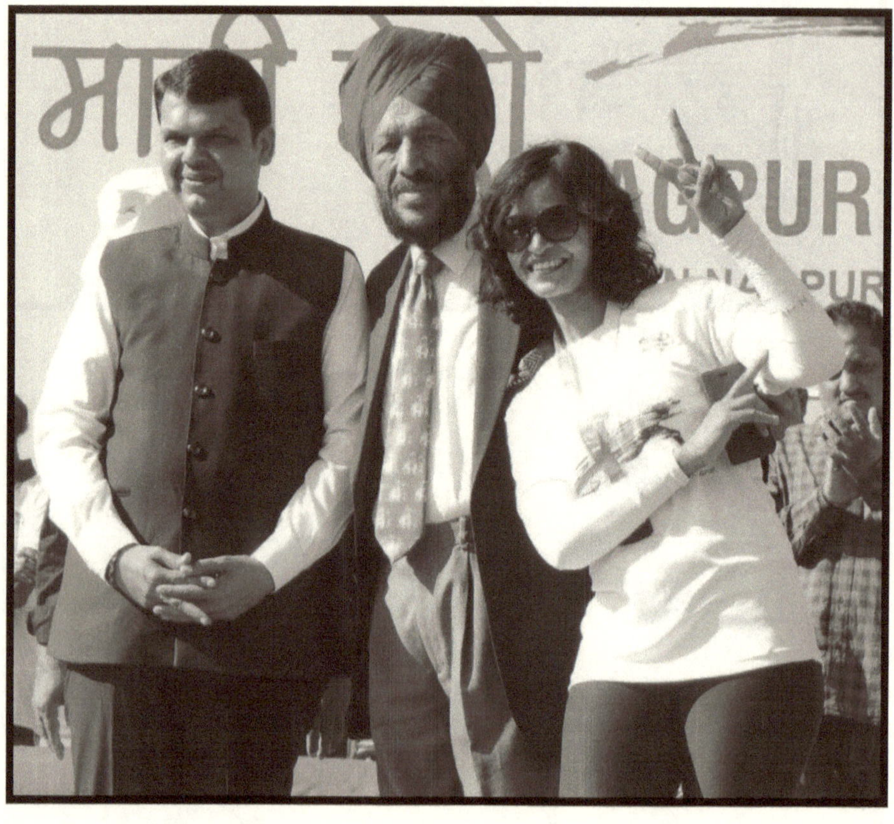

If You Want It, Go Get It | 10

Robotic Surgery Specialist, a Gynaec
Delivering Babies and a Tough IM Finisher

Dr. Ashwini, Mumbai

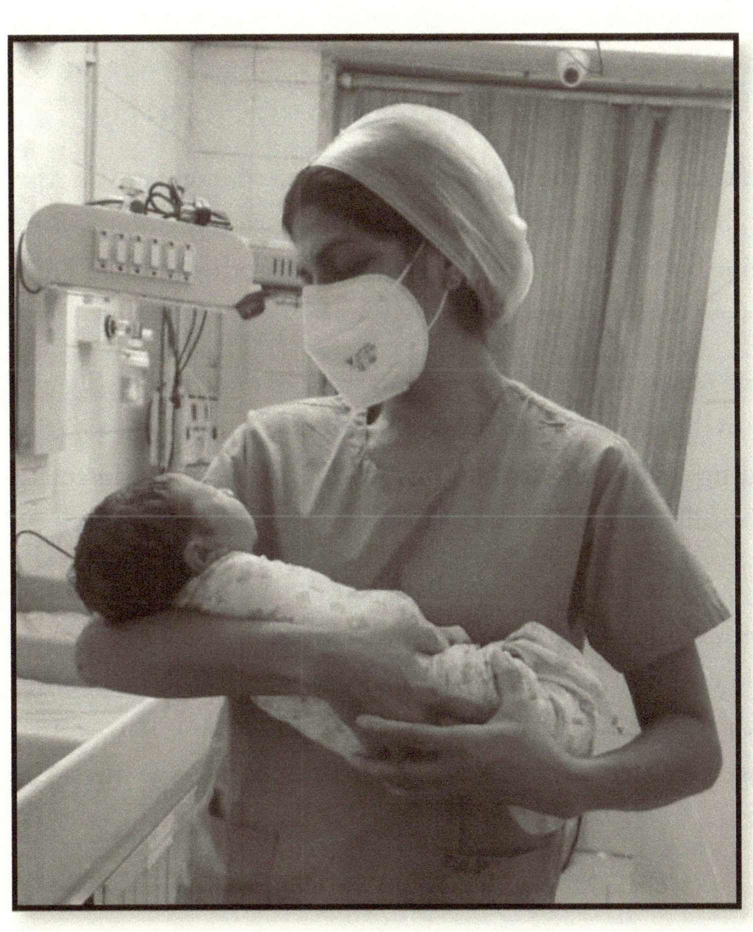

From being a nerdy student with the only aim to become a doctor to a practicing gynecologist to making tough choices for her family, 47-year-old Dr. Ashwini has come a long way – she's a podium finisher at the Kolhapur Triathlon, Turkey Ironman 70.3 finisher, and continues to race as she juggles her time between helping women deliver babies, training, two children, and more. Oh! Did we mention she performed Mumbai's first gynecological robot-assisted surgery?!

My Only Focus – Becoming a Doctor

I come from a Maharashtrian family where education was the utmost priority. My mother is a gynecologist, and I have seen her managing work and home with precision. I was always a sincere, *"accha-baccha"* (good kid), and was awarded the best student medal in grade 10.

My single focus was to be a gynecologist even though my mother warned me about the hard work followed by long working hours. But I was determined about my career goal. My elder brother went to KEM to become a gynecologist, and I followed his footsteps.

I played table tennis in my childhood but was never an athlete. Later, I loved going to the gym and was always fitness conscious. I went to KEM and enjoyed my tenure in learning medicine. I married my classmate, and I am blissfully married for 23 years now.

I started my private practice immediately after post-graduation, and I had no time for anything else. My kids were born in 2003 and 2006. I had multiple duties to address now. I had excellent live-in help, and I knew my babies were cared for well. Hence, I could focus on my work. I could manage breastfeeding by expressing milk to be given to my babies in my absence.

Life is a Series of Choices

My mother and mother-in-law both are working women, and I am proud to mention how beautifully they have managed their work-life balance. Although I had generous support that enabled me to focus on my career, due to long work hours, I could not attend to my kids as much as I would have wanted to.

When my daughter was ten months old, my full-time help left. I used to be in the clinic from 7–9 pm, and I returned home at 10 pm. I had to take a tough call. I had self-talk and concluded that my children would grow only once; my work will go on. I decided to manage my work timings according to their schedule and shifted my evening clinic hours to morning.

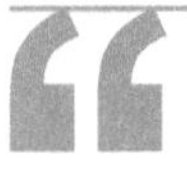

"There are choices to make at each point in life, but choose what makes you proud."

In 2011 two of my close friends did a half marathon, and the distance attracted me. The very next day, I was out in the neighboring park, trying to run. Not even 500 meters and I started panting, as I had run at full speed. An unknown lady who must have been 60 years of age was watching, and she approached me and asked if I aimed to run. She then offered to teach me and showed me how to run slowly and steadily without getting breathless. And I was then able to run 2 km efficiently.

I joined a running group called Run India Run. I did my first half marathon at SCMM (Standard Chartered Mumbai Marathon) under the able guidance of our excellent and inspiring Coach, Mr. Samson Sequeira.

I was in love with the outdoors now. We were blessed to train at Juhu beach, which is serene and beautiful in the early mornings. The morning training at the beach with constant encouragement and support from the rest of the group started on a positive and lively note.

In 2014 just a month before the SCMM, I incurred a stress fracture. I was extremely disheartened but I still went to the expo and collected the bib. I was restless the entire night before the race day, and seeing my state, my husband told me to go and run on the condition that I do not return further injured. I jumped out of the bed as if I was waiting for some push; I went ahead and finished the run.

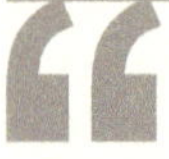

"Deep desires find their way."

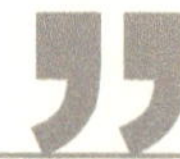

I then enrolled for 42 km. I developed hyperactive airways due to smog exposure in the winter months and had to take inhalers to be able to train. In two out of three full marathons that I attempted, I had bronchospasm despite the inhalers. I still completed the distance, though I wouldn't recommend anyone to do so, being a doctor myself. I realized that this was becoming counterproductive.

By this time, a couple of my friends had done the half Ironman, and the idea of doing three different sports back-to-back intrigued me. I decided to try it.

However, I had never trained in swimming. And I had hardly cycled in my childhood, and never after that. After the SCMM, I purchased a hybrid bike and enrolled for swimming lessons and enrolled for my first Duathlon at Vasai, where I stood fourth. I started learning to swim and cycle for races at the age of 45. After the Duathlon I attended a Tri camp to understand what a triathlon was all about. Most of the people there were experienced and talking about cadence, BRM, and other things, which were Greek to me. I felt out of place.

I joined swimming lessons keeping the Goa tri in mind, to be held in February 2018. Swimming and cycling were uphill tasks for me. I had to slog in the pool and put in lots of effort. In November, I tried to swim in a 50m pool and came out completely exhausted. Till November end, I was unable to swim 1500m in the pool. And here I was eyeing the Goa tri, where there was a sea swim! (quite ambitious).

I was determined to overcome this incompetency and gave it my best. And one beautiful November morning, some magic happened, and I could swim the pool's distance. I was amazed at this miracle. (Well, thinking about it later – it was my ardent effort of not giving up.)

Cycling was another challenge. I was terrified to ride on the road. I was scared of the traffic, potholes, being run over and of falls. It took me three years to finally think of cycling as fun. Before this, it was stressful for me. But with consistent practice, my strength grew. After completing the Goa tri, I registered for the Kolhapur triathlon in November 2018. I stood first in my age category and managed to shave off a good 30mins from my Goa timing.

For both Goa and Kolhapur triathlons, I trained under Dr. Kaustubh Radkar, and I thoroughly enjoyed the process. It was now time to take a plunge to the Ironman race. I registered for Turkey 70.3, and under the strict guidance of Viv Menon, I started my disciplined and structured training. Ashutosh Barve helped in a big way to improve my freestyle swimming.

The race in Turkey was a remarkable experience. The water was cold, and I struggled with headwinds during the bike course. But by God's grace, I completed all the three courses of swim, bike, and run successfully. All credit goes to Viv and Ashutosh for making me worthy of this medal.

It was a delight to see my family cheering for me at the finish line. I was genuinely grateful to complete the race, but I couldn't cherish the moment the way I had imagined it. My partner in crime, my best friend, with whom I had trained for all the races, had two punctures on the bike course and couldn't complete it. She was genuinely happy for me, though, and I hugged her with teary eyes. In our next race, I look forward to crossing the finish line together with her.

Managing the clinic, training hours, and children was challenging, but then it had to happen, so it did. I remember episodes when I have rushed to the clinic for emergency delivery calls and came back home to finish the remaining cycle training.

Learning at 45

There is learning in every race. I have grown from a person who didn't know swimming, was scared of cycling to a successful finisher in Turkey Ironman 70.3. I recall a childhood episode where I was in the pool with my cousin, splashing about at the shallow end. He jokingly dared me to jump into the pool's deep end (15 feet) from the first-floor diving board. Without hesitation, I went ahead and jumped. He was shocked and scared, as I didn't even know swimming. Giving-up and turning away from challenges doesn't come to me easily, I keep fighting until I attain my goal. This one incident pulled out the fear of open-water away from me.

Last year, I thought I would try to do the same thing. Now I knew swimming, and there was nothing to fear. But believe it or not, I walked to the edge of the first-floor board and couldn't muster the courage to jump! I turned back on two occasions. As children, we are far more fearless and daring than adults who are gripped in uncertainty and anxiety. Childhood experiences can translate into valuable life lessons. Skills like swimming and cycling when learned as a child remains for life.

I have also come across people who have labeled my race participation as a mid-life crisis. It is difficult to explain the finishing line's joy even when I haven't won the race.

"The more you explain, the more they will ask. Put your heart into your dreams; the questions will wither."

Be firm, stay firm and believe in yourself.

To All the Women Out there

Mother – As a mother, you'll always have unending responsibilities. You have to be the strongest pillar of the family. However, it is vital to find some me-time. Take care of yourself first to be a caregiver to others.

Gynecologist – Women need to do weight-bearing exercises, including strength training for better bone density. Strolls won't help to make bones stronger.

Please get back to the routine soon after childbirth. The best time to lose weight is during lactation when you can actually eat 500 calories extra and still lose weight if you exercise a bit. So start working out, and you'll be back in shape quickly.

Working woman – It is imperative for a woman to be financially independent, whether she needs to contribute to the household or not. A woman must have an income of her own. Children of working women are usually well adjusting, confident, and independent.

Athlete – Discipline, commitment and hard work, my training made me a better human being with lots of patience.

I can prioritize my work and other obligations.

I have started oil painting again and joined music classes too. My approach towards personal and professional life is more organized and structured.

Never think that you are too old to learn a new skill or start your journey on fitness. It all boils down to only one thing-

How badly do you want it, and how hard are you willing to work for it?

If you want, you will.

Take the plunge, and soon you'll be on the racing track!

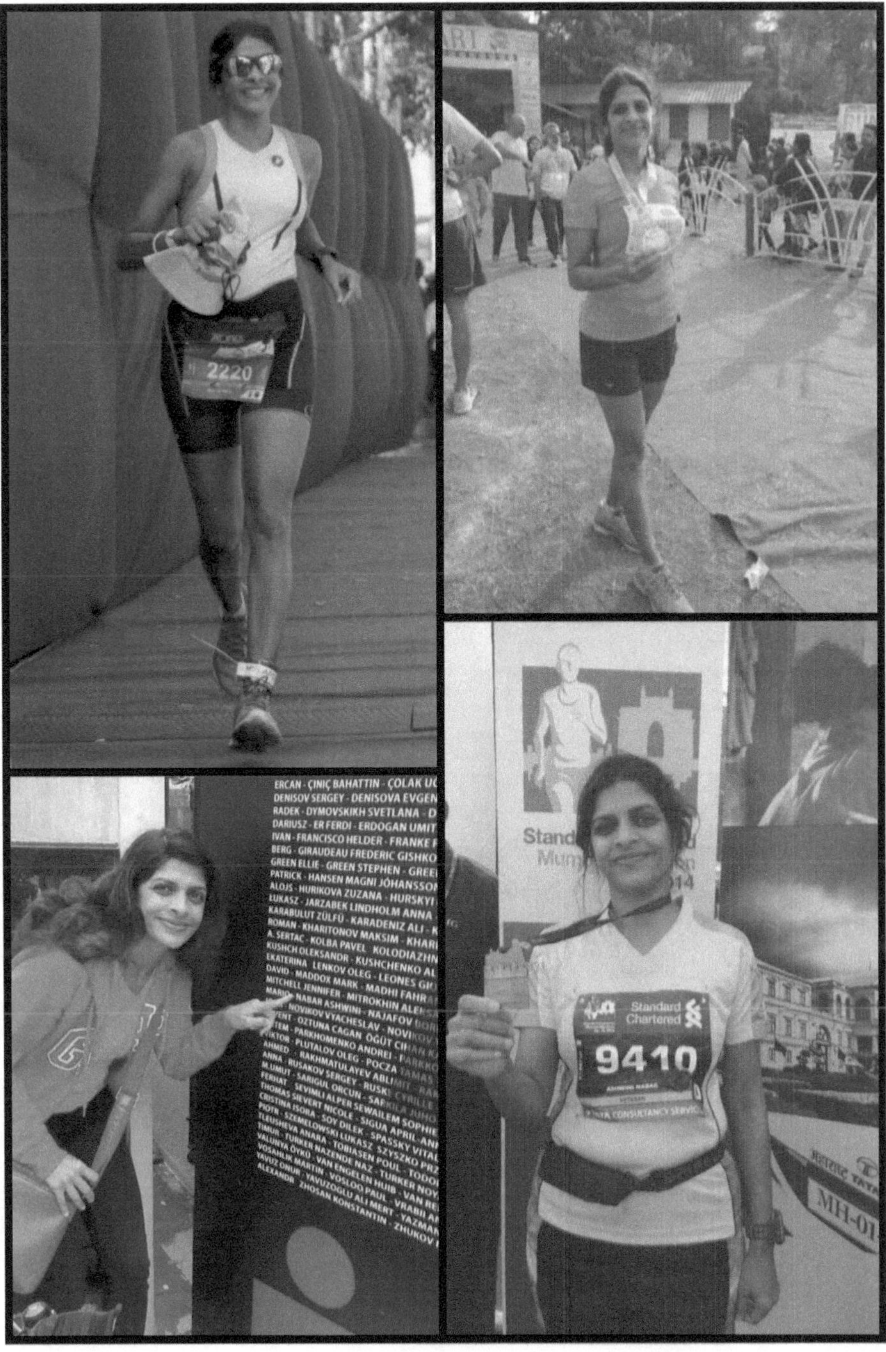

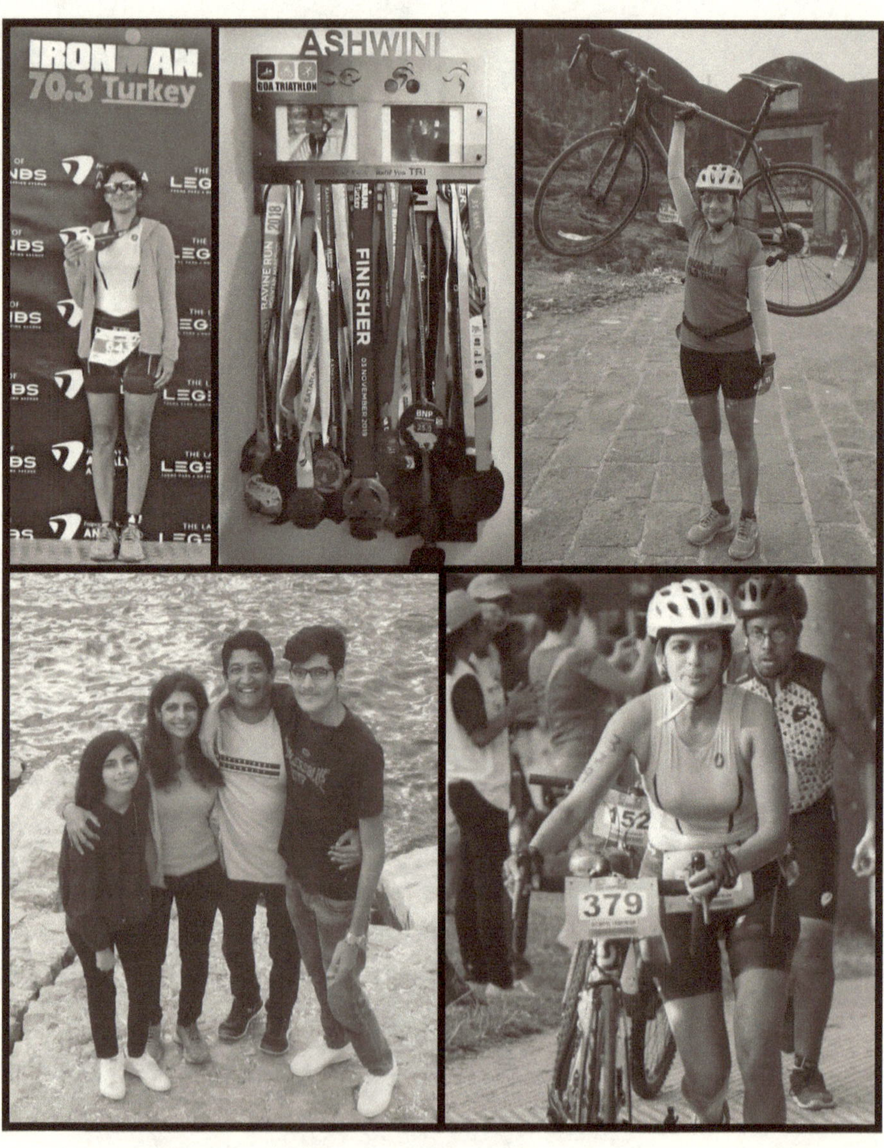
IRONMAN
70.3 Turkey
ASHWINI
GOA TRIATHLON
FINISHER
152
379

There is No Finish Line

Rest, Pause, Stop – What's That?

Anjali Bhalinge, Pune

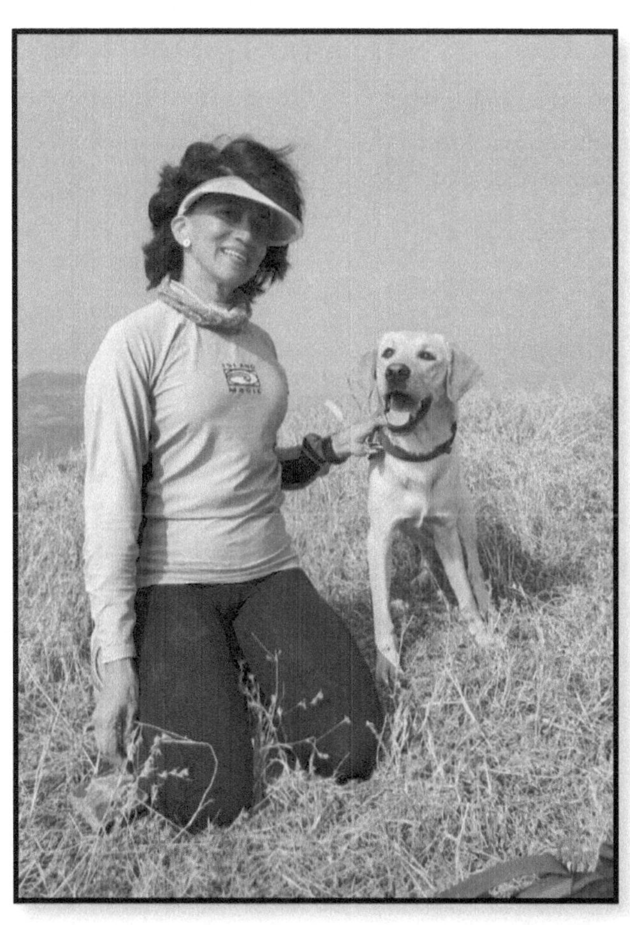

For most mothers, having two children with a not-so-satisfactory job and a home to run would mean giving up or settling for something mediocre, burying their dreams and aspirations, but not for Anjali Bhalinge. This 54-year-old Punekar goes full throttle at everything she does – Ironman, entrepreneurship, motherhood, family, and more.

Some of her achievements: Full Ironman – Vichy 2017, First rank in women's open category at Half Ironman Distance triathlon – Hyderabad 2015, First rank in Women's open category at Pune International 70.3 triathlon 2017, Second rank at Tata Ultramarathon 2019, third rank in 2020, podium finisher at several renowned cycling and running events like Mumbai marathon and Ahmedabad cyclothon, a podium finisher at TFN (Tour of Nilgiris) 2012, BMC (Basic Mountaineering Certification) A+ holder from NIM (Nehru Institute of Mountaineering), extreme adventure junkie, a non-believer of impossible, elite athlete, absolutely grounded human being, women entrepreneur, mother of two.

A Curious Childhood

My father was in the merchant navy. I've travelled far and wide with my family. Whenever the vessel ported, and my father got busy, my mother took us to explore the city.

I have seen my father extraordinarily fit and agile, hence I have always stayed fit and active. Fitness activities were a part of my lifestyle – swimming, cycling to school and then to college. I was a meritorious student and a SSC topper with second rank in Maharashtra. All my focus was on studies. Sports was nowhere on the radar. I think I am compensating now!

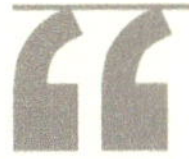

*"You manifest all your experiences of childhood
in your life. Ensure that you give the best to your
children too."*

Family vacations during our children's summer and winter breaks were a ritual. Even if my husband was busy at work and couldn't join us, I would take the girls for a holiday. Other than the family vacation, I also ensured that I take my solo trips either trekking, scuba diving, skiing, or any other adventure sport. I was not into spending on expensive clothes or buying my girls luxurious things. For me, it was more important to let my girls have travel experiences.

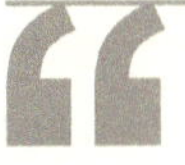

*"Blessed Are The Curious For They Shall Have
Adventures"*

Lovelle Drachman

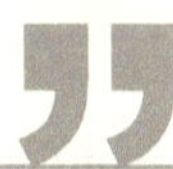

Shift, Hustle and the Discovery

Along with my engineering, I had pursued my passion for foreign languages – completing a diploma in Japanese language with 1st rank and a couple of courses in German too. I finished Engineering in 1988, got married, and my older daughter was born in 1991. I was working as a software professional with TCS but when I got a fantastic scholarship in 1992 to go to Japan on elective subjects, I chose Economics for wider learning experience. I finished the course and came back to India at the end of 1994.

Being in the software industry didn't entice me; hence I made a shift to a new job as a Japanese technical interpreter. It was a job that was not too creative and soon I got bored. I then worked with a firm to liaison with their Japanese counterpart, and there I got exposure to the export opportunities from India. In 1995, I finally plunged into entrepreneurship and started my own exports firm. A totally different world from my Engineering background – fabrics, fashion accessories and home decor!

By then my second daughter was born and life took a complete U-turn. Managing the new business, which required me to travel through the length and breadth of the country, to interior parts, as well as abroad to Japan, Chile and Argentina thrice a year. When I attempt something, I try to give it my best. For my South American customers, I attended a course in Spanish language. Doing all this and taking care of two young children with irregular work hours, I realized I was neglecting myself. Staying active was a lifestyle, hence I found some time late in the evening, after all my chores and got back to swimming. I swam religiously, irrespective of my impossibly hectic schedule.

In 2002, for my solo trip, I submitted the application for the Kailash Mansarovar yatra. I was thrilled to get the approval. This was not an easy trek, and it was mandatory to prepare well. Walking was never a part of my fitness journey. Sinhagad Fort is an excellent place to practise climbing, hence I started frequenting there very early in the morning.

This is where my fitness journey started. People say that the Kailash Mansarovar yatra is a life-changing experience, and it changed my life.

"Everyone wants to live on top of the mountain, but all the happiness and growth occurs while you are climbing it."

As preparation, I regularly started climbing Sinhagad Fort. I continued trekking it even after the Kailash yatra. All fitness enthusiasts frequent Sinhagad Fort as it gives a significant elevation as well all the training needed for any endurance race. It was here that I met people who not only inspired me but also encouraged and guided me at every point. I also got a sense of my potential, which I was unaware of.

During one of the weekly practices, I came across a group of gentlemen who were in their 60s and were planning to cycle from Goa to Cochin, which is more than 800 km. They asked me to join. Just the thought of trying it was petrifying, leave aside attempting.

When I showed reluctance, the gentleman from the group muttered a thought-provoking phrase, "Anything is possible if you practise and train." I started riding with them on my daughter's Miss India cycle, which, until then, I was using to run household errands. In 2004, I bought a bike for myself and cycled from Goa to Cochin with the group. I discovered myself.

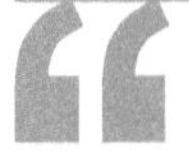

"The journey toward self-discovery is life's greatest adventure."

Arianna Huffington

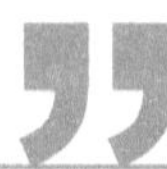

An Accidental Entry Into Racing

During one of the weekly Sinhagad climbs, I came across someone with a backpack, torch etc. I was curious and asked him about his gear. He told me that he traverses through forests at night to observe snakes, as he is a snake researcher. I was pleasantly surprised. He then asked me, "What do you do?"

"What do you do?" is a common question asked in our fitness enthusiast community. It has nothing to do with socio-economic status, but it means, "What other physical activity do you do?"

I told him that I cycle and swim a bit. He offered to ride together. I gladly agreed. After the ride, he suggested that I should join the Pune cycling team. My jaws dropped in amazement at his suggestion. I was in my 40s and getting into an elite team was beyond my vision.

I respected his suggestion as he was an ex-bicycle-racer and might have seen some potential in me. I got a road bike and participated in the trials for the Pune team. I was among the first four to finish and then also got selected for the Maharashtra team standing along with girls my daughters' age!

In 2006, on one of the sinhagad hikes, a fellow enthusiast asked me if I ran too as he saw me climbing fast. He asked me to join for the half marathon training. I was zapped knowing the distance but decided to give it a try. Coincidently, my mother gifted me a Labrador puppy around that time and then it became a ritual to run with her every morning. My dog Elle was my running partner and that's how my running started.

In 2007, I participated in the Mumbai Marathon and stood third in my first half marathon. I was extremely happy for myself. Thus, I started my racing journey, and somehow, I grabbed the podiums in most of the races.

"Good health, peace of mind, being outdoors, camaraderie: those are all wonderful things that come to you when running. But for me, the real pull of running—the proverbial icing on the cake—has always been racing."

To Triathlons

Whenever I look back, I realize that my triathlon journey started right from my childhood. I was swimming, cycling and even running; it was not for any event, but I was doing it on my own and unknowingly building up on stamina as well. I thought of participating in a triathlon much earlier, but somehow it didn't work out. I have a firm belief that when things have to happen, they will, so go with the flow.

Meanwhile, I participated in Enduro (a high-paced multi discipline adventure race held in Pune). The event used to last for two days, and in a team of three, one participant has to be a female. It is a self-supported event where we have to ride off-road, carry our bikes, climb a steep hill, rappel down a cliff, cross a river and few other things. The race is a test of stamina and team coordination. I participated in this event for two consecutive years, and after getting a podium in the first year, my team finally emerged as winners in the second year.

My stamina increased substantially due to my gradual progress in all the sports. I participated in TFN (Tour of Nilgiris) and was a podium finisher in 2012. I also participated many times in the Tour of Tamilnadu which is a cycling picnic tour exploring the beauty of Tamil Nadu.

Finally, I participated in my first triathlon – the half Ironman distance 70.3 triathlon, Hyderabad in 2015 after a friend who had already done 15 then (now over 25) Ironman persuaded me to do it. I stood first in the women's open category. Swimming in open waters was never a fear as I've seen the sea up close since my childhood and I am also a certified scuba diver. I was now keen to do a full Ironman. Once I attain a level, I want to raise the bar higher.

Meanwhile, I kept gathering podiums in marathons and other races. Somehow the podiums fall in my kitty – strange!

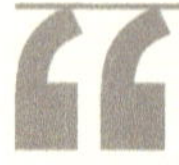

> *"I also realize that winning doesn't always mean getting first place; it means getting the best out of yourself."*
>
> *Meb Keflezighi, 2004 Olympic Marathon silver medalist*

In 2016, I broke my shoulder bone and went on a pause-mode for a while. In 2017, I participated in Full Ironman, Vichy, France and gracefully completed the race. It was beautiful to see my family at the finish line. My daughter was in the US at that time and came to France to cheer me on. This race was a gift to myself on my 50th birthday. The biggest celebration was to cross the finish line. My type of partying!

Year	Event
2002	Kailash Mansarovar
2004	Goa-Cochin cycling ride
2007	Mumbai Marathon (third position)
2012	TFN (Tour Of Nilgiris), podium finisher in race segment
2013	Enduro race, winner team
2015	Hyderabad 70.3(first position in women's open category)
2017	Full Ironman, Vichy
2019	Basic Mountaineering Course from Nehru Institute of Mountaineering
2019	Cycling Imphal to Bangkok via Myanmar
2019	Boston qualifier at Chicago
2019	RAAM qualifier Shivalik Signature, Chandigarh
2020	TMM (Tata Mumbai Marathon), Boston qualifier 3:49:20
2020	Hiranandani Half marathon, winner in age category
2020	Tata Ultra, podium in age category
2020	Hall of fame of Everesting, completed Ride half Everesting(base camp)
2021	Hall of Fame of Everesting, Completed Ride 10k Everesting, at present the oldest Indian to do this.

Conquering Fear

It was in 2012, during the Enduro Race that I came face to face with acrophobia. The race had a condition that the rappling should be done by the female participant only. It was a nerve wrenching task for me. I had to overcome this fear.

Fast forward to 2018, battling my fear. I came across a young guy during my fitness journey. During one conversation, he told me that he was a trekker and aimed to be a mountaineer. He was soon to do a course in basic mountaineering from the Nehru Institute of Mountaineering. I was excited to hear this, but my excitement faded quickly. He informed me that the age limit was 40 years, and I was way beyond the age limit.

I was determined to do the course and called up the Principal at NIM. I requested him to accommodate me; I showed him my keenness and also told him about my accomplishments.

He hanged the call asking me to drop a mail. It was a clear sign that nothing would materialize.

In 2019, just out of curiosity, I called up the Principal again, and he was surprised that he hadn't received my request mail. I was disappointed. But then he asked me to check the website for the eligibility criteria. I checked; they had modified the age limit to 55 years.

He didn't just make alterations for the age limit but also accommodated me in the immediate mixed batch of the Basic Mountaineering Course. I was indeed the oldest in the group but awarded the best cadet. The tough training helped me overcome acrophobia.

Things happen, the universe conspires, don't give up and keep trying.

The American civil rights leader, Susan B Anthony, wrote in 1896: *"I think (the bicycle) has done more to emancipate women than any one thing in the world. I rejoice every time I see a woman ride by on a bike. It gives her a feeling of self-reliance and independence the moment she takes her seat; and always she goes, the picture of untrammelled womanhood."*

With this belief, in November 2019, I did a cycle ride along with a few friends where we rode to Bangkok travelling across three countries, Imphal to Bangkok via Myanmar. I feel more connected with nature and self when I am on my bike. I also noticed that after the lockdown was lifted, the housemaids who had bicycles, were the first ones to resume work. Cycling is freedom.

With the lack of races during the lockdown, to keep the training going, Everesting became the latest fad. And India is not far behind. Everesting involves picking a hill anywhere in the world and riding repeats of it in a single activity until you climb 8,848 m – no walking and no sleeping. It is crazy. And in this act of madness, I went beyond Everesting (8,848 metres), to do the 10K Ride Everesting. I am officially in the Everesting Hall of Fame and as of now I am the oldest Indian to do the 10k ride Everesting.

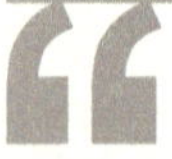

"It always seems impossible until it's done."

Nelson Mandela

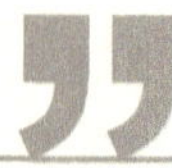

March Ahead

I started with racing events pretty late in life. I didn't get a coach for the training because I wasn't preparing for any race. My training had actually started during my childhood, where I was exposed to all aspects of travel, life, sports and endurance. I wasn't even aware, but I was building myself one step at a time. When the events started happening, I was already prepared and gave in my best.

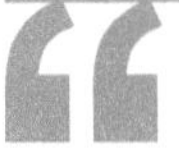

"The more difficult the victory, the greater the happiness in winning."

Pele

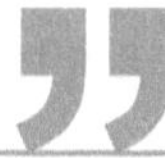

For anyone who is preparing for any race, don't get into high-paced training. Give yourself time, let your body pick up bits and pieces, build upon your stamina, get along with like-minded people, people who motivate and encourage you at every point, give in your best as there are no shortcuts to success.

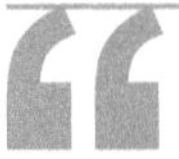

"If you fall behind, run faster. Never give up, never surrender, and rise up against the odds."

Jesse Jackson

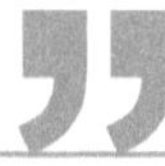

As a mother of two, I never lost myself in duties and responsibilities. Today when I see my daughters grown up as strong independent young girls, making their own decisions, I feel proud for being a tough and independent mother. They've seen a mother who lives by her terms and has a go-getter spirit. If you want to raise strong-headed children, then be strong, very strong and keep marching ahead.

> *"Courage, sacrifice, determination, commitment,*
> *toughness, heart, talent, guts. That's what little girls*
> *are made of; the heck with sugar and spice."*
>
> **Bethany Hamilton**

At the age of 54, this little girl asks all the ladies to move out and create that hustle – trust me, you won't regret it.

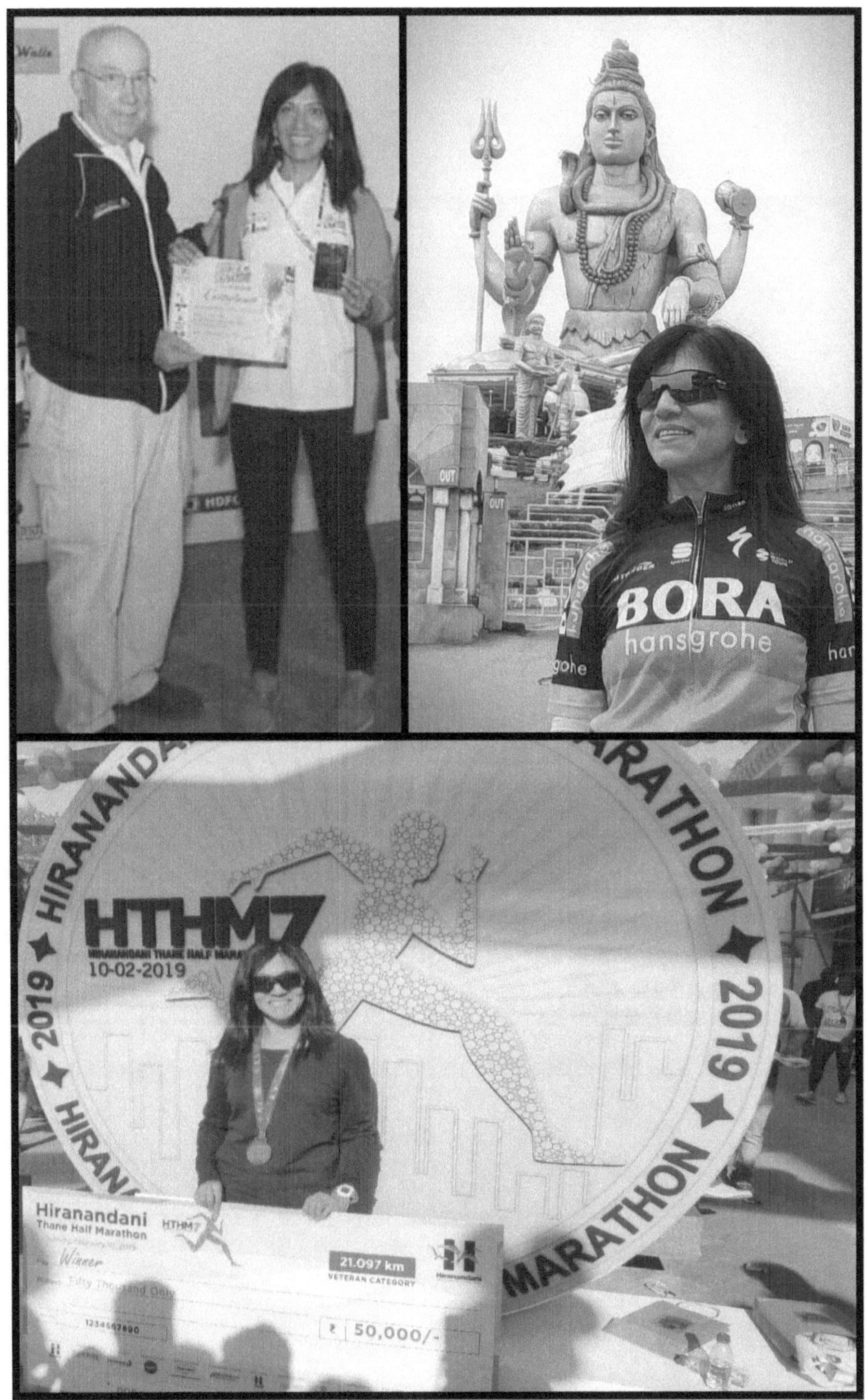
BORA
hansgrohe
2019
HIRANANDANI
MARATHON
HTHM7
10-02-2019
2019
Hiranandani
Thane Half Marathon
Winner
21.097 km
VETERAN CATEGORY
₹ 50,000/-
1234567890

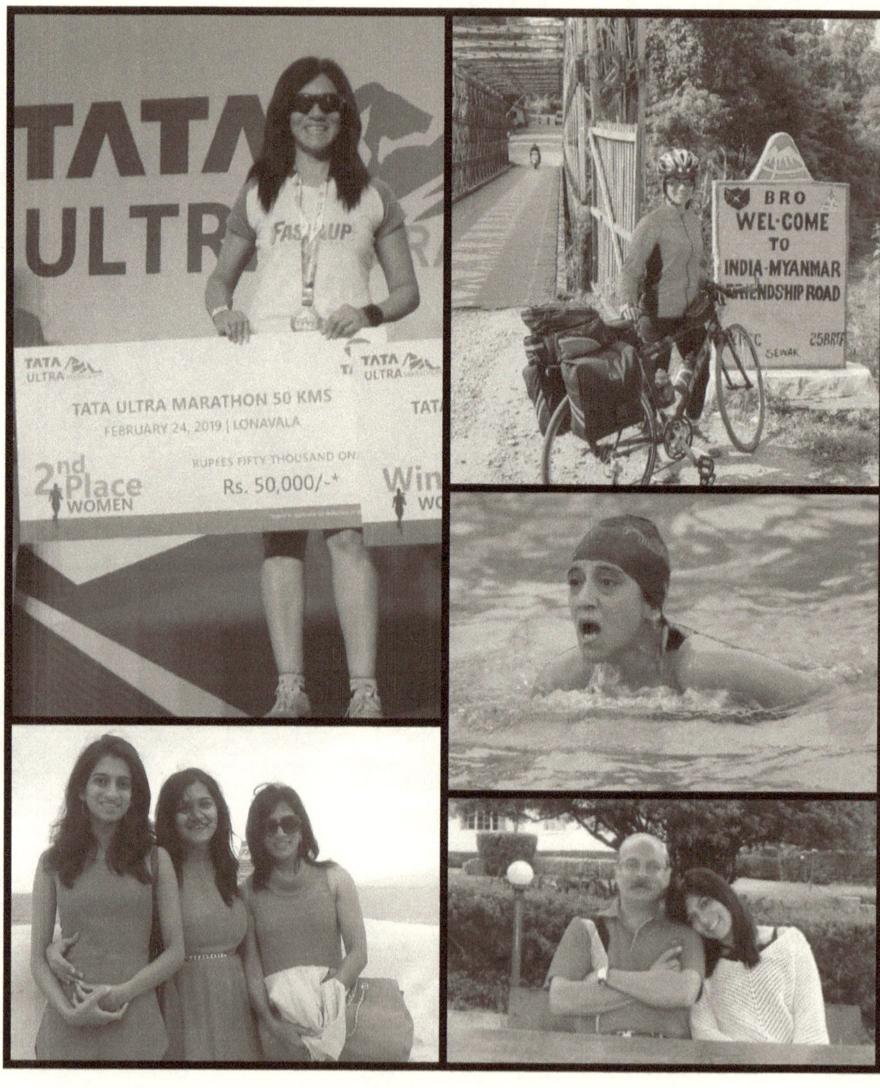
TATA
ULTRA
TATA ULTRA MARATHON 50 KMS
FEBRUARY 24, 2019 | LONAVALA
RUPEES FIFTY THOUSAND ON
2nd Place WOMEN
Rs. 50,000/-*
BRO
WEL·COME
TO
INDIA-MYANMAR
FRIENDSHIP ROAD

Hurt? So What, Get Up and Start All Over Again

Crash Queen

Chandani Desai, Dubai

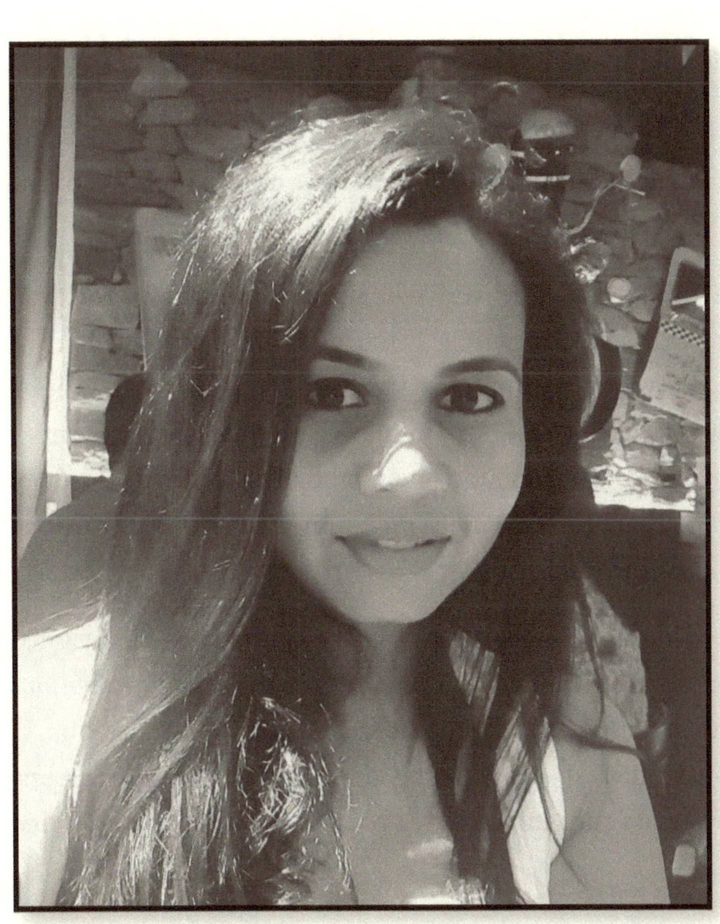

Just like the waves in the sea come crashing to the shore but never do they stop – somewhat similar is Chandani Desai. A thyroid patient, mother of a nine-year-old, textile designer, she calls herself 'Crash Queen'. Every time she gets on her bike, she crashes, but that doesn't crash her spirit. She keeps picking up herself and pedaling on.

Like a Soldier in a Battlefield

There hasn't been any race where I haven't fallen off my bike. My knees are forever bleeding, injured, bandaged, and bruised. After every race, I look like a wounded soldier just returned from the battlefield. Now, I've come to a consensus that crashing is a good omen for me.

I come from a family where outdoor explorations like treks, hikes, and long walks were regular affairs. While my family post-marriage was the opposite, my husband would not prefer going out at all, gradually, I also got pulled into married life responsibilities. I was never a high adrenaline person, but I was fit and agile. I was juggling multiple things.

There came a moment post-delivery when I could not get off the floor without support. It was demeaning. I didn't like my state. But I didn't know what to do. When my son started his play-school in the afternoon shift, I managed to find 45 minutes in between his drop and pick up. I used this time to run, at 12noon, come rain, hail or shine. I used to go home, shower, prepare his tiffin, and pick him up. Whenever I missed the run, I climbed the stairs.

My building residents thought that I was crazy. Yes, I madly wanted to get back to my fit-form and not remain a slug. I was synonymous with Mumbai express, on time, can't get slow, will never stop. I could now run around 10 km, but the city-run was boring. Someone mentioned the Satara run. In no time, I registered and finished my first half marathon.

Some People Crib, Some Join the Madness

In 2013, my husband, Pratik, did his first Comrades. Due to several reasons, he broke his spine and was on complete bed rest. His first question to the doctor was – will I be able to run? Running is his life, and he was slipping into depression due to his injury.

I had to take a call here to crib about his state or join him in his madness. I chose the latter, and that is how my events journey started. We started sharing a lot of things in common. I could now relate to the jargons used in training. As I juggled between a kid, work, home, and more, he understood my pain points and started supporting me even more. I could now extract time from my schedule and train devotedly.

Bitten By the Tri-bug

In 2016, I got to know about the Pune Triathlon. Running was getting boring, and the combination of three sports seemed attractive. I registered for the event and started training.

My schedule was something like this:

➤ Wake up at 5 am and go for training

➤ Cook breakfast, lunch for the whole family

➤ Get Rivaan ready for school

➤ Take the train to work (missing a local in Mumbai is like missing your work)

➤ Leave on time from work

➤ Pick up Rivaan, drop him to classes

➤ Cook dinner

➤ Train once everyone in the house is asleep

I was running on a reserve battery. I used to get super tired, drained out, but I found myself more energetic than I was earlier because first, I was enjoying the pain, and second it was a feel-good factor. Pratik came forward to take care of Rivaan and encouraged me to train harder for my first triathlon, which later got him hooked as well.

I came to know about my naive state when, during one cycle training session, I tried hard to catch up with my co-trainee, but my cycle wouldn't move forward at all, no matter how hard I tried. He then offered his bike, and I realized the difference between an autorickshaw and a Ferrari.

The race day was also disastrous. I lost my way during the swim course and swam a half Ironman distance (1.9 km) compared to the Olympic (1.5 km). I was screaming mid-way to guide me for the direction. A kind soul heard me and shouted back to swim 45 degrees right. I swam in my swimming costume and just wore a cycling tee over it for the bike course. The concept of wet suit or any other gear was unknown until then.

The bike course was not just tough but grueling. It was on the ghats, and I had trained only on the plains. Anyhow, I patted myself that I completed the course without a fall. But this happiness was short-lived, and I crashed, yet again.

The last running course was the toughest. I had cramps in my legs right from the start. One person told me to have salt at the station, another told me to have gel. I did what I could, and dragged myself.

In the last 200 meters where I was still pushing myself, Pratik cheered me loudly, "Go run, the medal is yours. You have only two minutes left". I composed myself, pushed as hard as I could, and crossed the finish line. I sat there and cried my heart out. Those were the tears of my hard work, discipline, my express routine, Pratik's injury, my child who saw me training hard, and all my effort. I deserve this medal, yes, the medal was mine!

Going For 70.3

In 2017, Pratik and I did the Pune International Triathlon together (It was his first and my second), and the same year we shifted to Dubai. Fast forward to 2018, while I was still adjusting to the new country, work, and Rivaan's school, Pratik completed his first 70.3 and went to do his first full at IM Hamburg. It is here, while cheering for him and seeing him cross the red carpet that I got goosebumps and a thought flashed in my mind to do Dubai 70.3 along with him.

My thought turned into reality in India when we went to meet the only Iron couple Kaushik and Vineeta over a weekend drink. Within a second of sharing my thoughts about doing an Ironman, they registered me for Dubai 70.3, and then there was no looking back!

Mis(s)adventures

With the event approaching, I had lots to catch up and get into aggressive training. The training period was strenuous. Being a slow racer and also a thyroid patient, my recovery rate is more time-consuming. My legs would ache to give me sleepless nights. Rivaan used to sit on my legs to comfort me, but every single day, I would wake up with the same zeal and train much harder than the previous day.

On my first-century training ride (100 km), after 18 km, I had a crash (nothing new in that), but this time my cycle didn't move no matter how hard I pedaled. I kept going and finished the ride. I then called up Pratik to pick me up as I was almost immobile. I started worrying about my capability to finish the bike course in the race. When Pratik came to pick me up and had a look at the bike and me, he sensed my worry.

With a smile on his face, he assured me that I was more than ready for the race. I was puzzled. He told me that the brakes jammed after the crash, and even then, I completed the ride. This effort talked a lot about my stamina and strength. I was confident about biking now.

Then came the swim struggle. I was excellent at breaststroke, but it wasn't easy in a wetsuit. I changed to freestyle just three weeks before the race. Also developed severe bronchitis. On the race day, I entered the water with bruised knees and cuts so deep that the flesh was visible—courtesy-all the falls during the training.

The water was choppy, but I managed to finish the swim course. My Garmin malfunctioned on the event day, and I was unwary of the time. I got on the bike, and as always, a fall had to happen. I got back on the bike and completed the bike course as well. The run was draining.

I panicked because of the time. Pratik passed on the message that I had time to finish. I was relieved to hear that, but I was exhausted. I saw people older than me running to the finish line, and I silently muttered to myself – you will not give up Chandani, run, go, run to the finish line. As soon as I saw the red carpet, I sprinted and finished well before time.

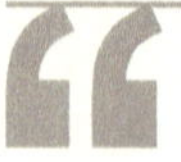
"Firm your mind, and the universe will conspire to make it happen."
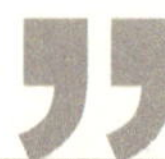

Pick Up, pedal Up

I had to come over challenging circumstances for all my races, but I was a tougher challenge. I was determined, and one after the other, things kept falling in place to train systematically. Crashing is my second name, but I never gave up and carried on with bleeding knees in all the races even then. Just recently, entirely, out of nowhere, I had a massive crash in a casual bike ride during the lockdown. I had to undergo facial surgery with multiple fractures. It was a tough time to manage in a foreign country and a child back home. He was petrified to see my injured face. Two months post-surgery, I am back on the saddle again.

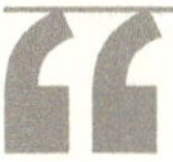

"There will be challenges and setbacks in some way or the other; sit back or get going — the choice is yours."

To All You Women

We, women, are crash queens in our ways.

Stereotypes can crash us

Heaps of responsibilities can crash us

Guilt can crash us

But we have to rise and shine for we are the queens

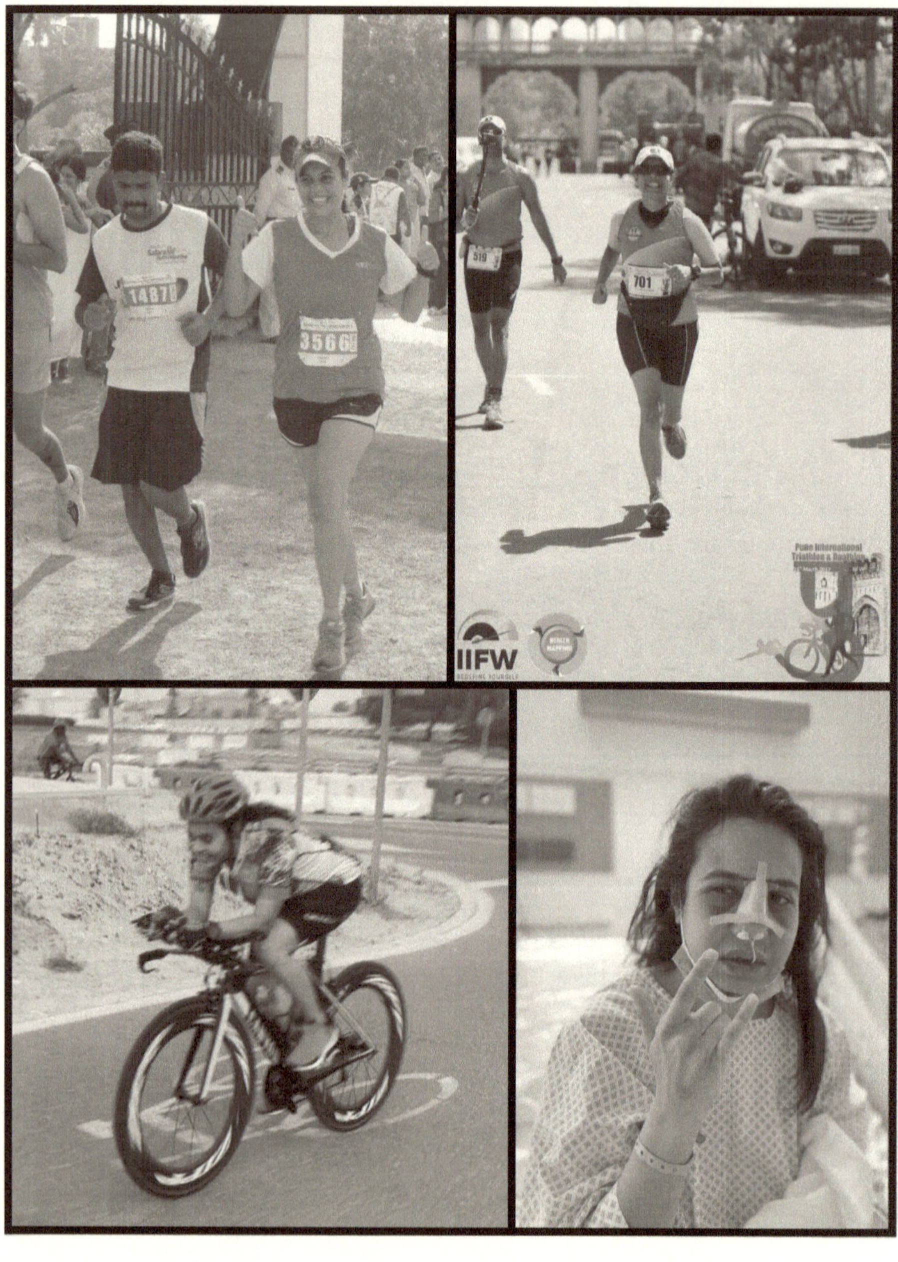

You Are Your Own Limit 13

Tough, Bold and Beautiful

Preeti Mohan, Singapore

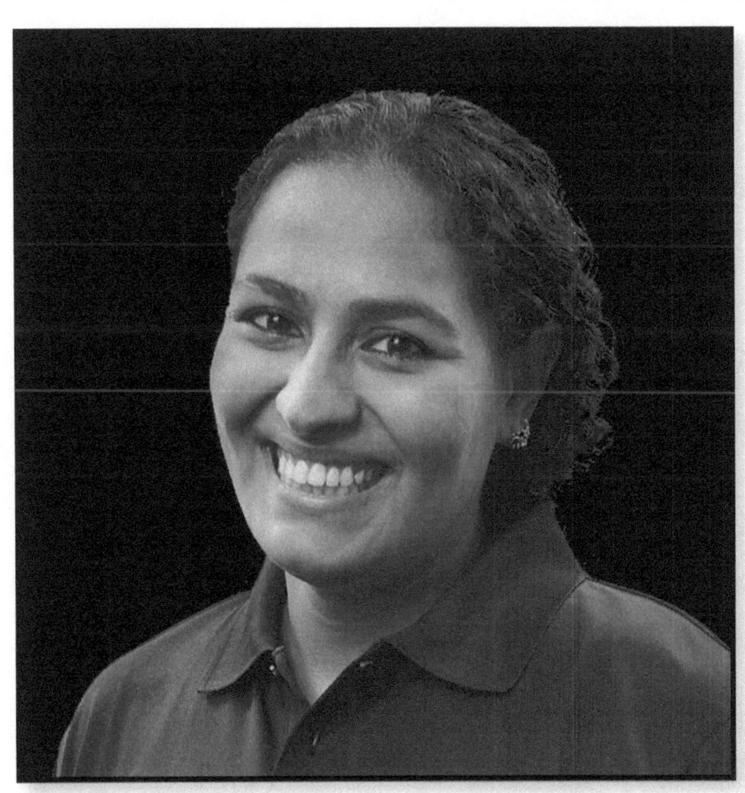

Bruised, abused, uprooted from her comfort surroundings, overweight at one point, 38-year old Preeti Mohan is now a biomedical engineer, start-up woman, a bharatnatyam dancer, finisher of over 40 races in seven years including Danang 70.3 in 2017, Bintan 70.3 in 2017, Davao 70.3 2018, Kapas Marang 6.5K swimathon in 2018, Ironman Malaysia (DNF) in 2018, a lady with an ever-smiling face, a generous heart to help, one of the brainchild behind the Facebook community for Indian Women Triathletes, mother of two lovely boys. And going by her aspirations, she's just getting started.

Bruised, Abused, Not Beaten

I was born in Chennai, brought up in Mumbai and grew up in Singapore. I think I was born with a passion for dancing; my parents tell me I started dancing at the age of two just watching the television. I formally started learning Indian classical dance when I was three years old. I didn't play any sport beyond physical education in school. My weekends usually revolved around dance rehearsals and performances from a young age. I loved it, dance taught me discipline and passion. It allowed me to express myself in a way I truly enjoyed.

I was also a very active child; I would climb everywhere and jump from all sorts of heights. Trees, trucks, buildings, what not! I fractured my foot many times because of this. My mom says she cannot remember a day I didn't come home bruised.

In 1992, to have a better and secure future, my parents abruptly migrated to Singapore. It was the most challenging phase of my life. My stage shows stopped; dancing came to a standstill. I was my grandparents' pet, and I missed them a lot; above all, I didn't have any friends. I had to cope with a completely new culture and system. I went from being a spoilt, carefree child to needing to become a responsible "teenager"

(I was only 11), almost immediately. Initially, my father didn't have a job in Singapore, while mom worked night shifts at a factory. Then as things settled, dad got a job and used to travel a lot. Mom picked up a career as a teacher. Finances were tight and my parents worked really hard. We had to be frugal about everything.

Things were tough then. My mom would work all day and study in the evenings, so she would leave early and come back home late. My brother and I were mostly on our own after school, and we readily participated in our parents' struggle. My father was proactive in all the housework, and we all had designated chores. I faced a lot of racism in the school where kids would make fun of my complexion, body type, hair or even the shape of my eyes. I had no friends to play with, neither in school, nor in the neighborhood.

My teenage years were probably the toughest for me. It was around this time that a priest who befriended my mother in the temple started sexually abusing me at my own home. He would visit in the pretence of seeing my mother. She had recently lost her father and saw a father figure in him. I had no friends and the situation in my house was such that I couldn't tell my parents what was happening. No matter how hard I tried to avoid him, he would still manage to get me alone. He even sexually assaulted me in the temple a few times. I totally lost faith in religion, God, and myself. I was petrified and confused. I couldn't bring myself to share it with my parents, they had enough going on already.

After a few months my perpetrator left Singapore, but my self-confidence had plummeted by then. I hated my body. I felt unclean and ashamed of it. I was sinking into the dark with suicidal thoughts. So often I would just think of jumping off from a building and just ending my life. I started eating out of anxiety, I would wear baggy clothes and wished I wasn't a girl. I hated taking photos or looking at myself in the mirror. I had massive trust issues with regards to people, especially men.

I had a distinct change in my behaviour. I became guarded from anyone and everyone around, and I went into my shell, and my aggression was visible too. Banging doors, screaming, tantrums, were a few coping mechanisms.

Finally, after four years, I mustered courage and shared the ordeal with my parents. My parents were soothingly supportive and took the situation in their stride. I started setting goals for myself and started working towards them. It was only in junior college and university that I made some really good friends. They changed my perspective about men, not all men are bad.

Around this time, I am grateful I met my dance teacher, my *mami* (aunt), who took me under her wings. She helped me find my outlet in dance again and it became a way of expression for me. It was my escape, my get away from this world. I could go to dance class and be whoever I wanted to be. I plunged myself into more dancing, to an unhealthy level. At times, I would dance for hours, pushing my past injuries and kept dancing. It became an obsession. So often after a performance, my friends would literally carry me home because my ankle ligament would tear on stage and I didn't even realise. It was around this time I started swimming breaststroke (the only stroke I knew) for recovery of my ankle injuries.

One night I was walking alone around my university and a drunken worker staggered towards me and caught me. It was a terrible struggle for me to escape and run back to my room. Sadly, that brought back all the sleeping demons. I would see imaginary people in my room and scream in the middle of the night, I had a lot of panic attacks. Thankfully this time my friends came to my rescue and really helped me through that phase. Overtime, I started travelling more avidly and backpacked across many countries, even did a solo trip to Europe, overcoming many of my fears and trust issues.

Fast forward to 2006, Sumit, my husband, came in quite suddenly into my life and swept me off my feet. He helped me to truly heal from my past to a point where I can talk about what happened. He provided me a safe space of trust.

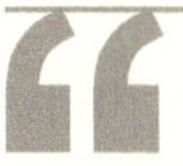

> *He has shown me that a good relationship is not about compromise only but also about helping each other grow to achieve more.*

The First High

I delivered my first child in 2011. I had a safe pregnancy and was looking forward to a new experience; little did I know about the aftermath. I developed a few complications before and after the delivery like symphysis pubis dysfunction (SPD), placenta previa, pre-eclampsia and finally shingles (on the day I delivered). Due to shingles, my entire face swelled up, and I could not open my eyes to see my baby and feed. Like any other first-time mother, I had my own set of nervousness and anxiety. It was a challenging phase as more than the infant I had to manage myself. My husband and mother-in-law became my strongest pillars of support. She would comfort and soothe me as she was worried that I would slip into postpartum depression. After the initial six-months of the difficult time, things started settling in, and I turned into a huge mommy with a whopping 90kgs in my kitty!

I started working out daily, long walks and strength work. Although I lost 18kgs in one and a half years, my husband made a valid point – how will you sustain this weight loss? He suggested that I look up for a few races or events that will keep me motivated. In 2013, I signed up for TriYas 2014 and found the race pattern pretty interesting. I had never attempted a triathlon before and wasn't even aware of the format.

Even then, I was too enthusiastic and was looking forward to the event. I realised for someone who had never been into sports, I had only six months to prepare. I was very diligent – did a lot of research online and learnt as much as I could find. But I didn't know anyone who had done triathlons, to reach out and ask.

I got my first mountain bike worth 150 Dirhams and was beaming with joy. Until now I was swimming breaststroke in the pool, but on race day I had to swim in the sea, hence, I decided to try out swimming in the ocean. So I ventured into the sea on my own. I could only go in till the water touched my ankle. In the chilly winters of November to December 2013, it was a routine that after dropping my son to the playschool and finishing the necessary chores, I would go to the beach at 10am and venture two inches further in the sea. Finally, in January, I could do two to three loops (race was in Feb). Whenever I went to the sea, I was always a single one practising, moreover struggling with the waves, and jumping at every twig that touched me.

Venturing on my own without worrying about what will happen next is my childhood trait. Back in Singapore, after my school got over, I would board random buses and go around the city. Sometimes I got lost too, and that was the time my mother caught my mischief. I did a similar thing in Mumbai when I was seven years old. I had a dance rehearsal, and due to some communication gap, my teacher was late to pick me up. I went on my own to the centre from Kings' Circle to Andheri, changing two trains and a bus, leaving everyone stunned.

I was unsure about the race, but now that I had registered and invested a lot of time and money, I headed to collect the bib. The race environment was electrifying. I was like a lamb in a slaughterhouse. Athletes of all build and form surrounded me. I meekly collected my kit and bumped into Smita. Ah! what a relief to meet a fellow Indian woman at the race.

On the race day, Sumit and my two and a half-year-old son accompanied me. It was an evening race and just after an hour of reaching the venue, my son started running a high temperature. I was in split minds to attempt the race or not. Sumit, my rock, encouraged me to go ahead and race.

The event was held in the marina area, and I made a mistake to slide down for a swim than jumping into the water, scraping my feet against the uneven wall. No sooner I was in the water, my foot started burning, and as if that was not enough, someone knocked off my goggles. At 300 meters, I held on to the kayak, composed myself and started swimming again. I was the last one to finish the swim course. I then changed into track pants and tee for the bike course (now when I think about this, I feel amused). I was riding my mountain for a triathlon, and I was on cloud nine as the cycling course was on the F1 racing track. Where on earth will I ever get a chance to ride my bike in this beautiful arena? I loved the experience.

When I came to my bike, everyone else was packing and going, but then I heard volunteers cheering – "give way, biker coming!" I was thrilled as I was probably the last one, yet everyone was cheering. That's the spirit that attracted me to this community.

The bruises from the scrape were hurting with each step of the run and I was among the last two to finish the race. I was not bothered that the banner was pulled off when I reached the finish line, but I was thrilled to see my supporters (Sumit, my son Pranav, Smita and her husband, Suk, and another family friend) cheering for me. I had a euphoric finish.

Smita and I signed up for Abu Dhabi International coming up in two weeks, and in all enthusiasm, we trained together and completed that race too. My journey in tri had started, and I was indeed not looking back.

Races and Some More Races

I had my second boy in July 2015, he was a child born with many issues but within four months I was back to cycling at 4am. It was my escape, my alone time to cope with the rest of the day. I completed the TriYas and ITU event in 2016, and then we unexpectedly moved to Singapore.

I was back to dancing and working in the hospital. My parents helped me a lot with managing my kids while I trained, which usually happened when my kids slept. The athletics community was not the same as Abu Dhabi. People were super competitive. If someone was a slow racer, then even the attempt to race was questionable. At that time there were hardly any women in the training groups or multisport races. But unlike UAE, races happened in plenty and throughout the year.

I learnt how to swim freestyle properly and took part in many rides and runs. I was also able to try many new formats of multisport including RunSwimRun, SwimRunSwim, etc. I was loving it and I wanted more! I was on a racing high and did almost 20 races in 2016–17 including Ironman Danang 70.3 and Bintan 70.3 in 2017.

In 2018 I decided to take on the full Ironman and started training for it. I participated in a variety of races to build upon endurance, including Davao 70.3, Kapas Marang 6.5 km swim in Malaysia where we had to swim from one island to the other, NTU Bike Rally – 180km, few half marathons etc. However, I DNFed at Bintan 70.3 2018 in August and the Tour de Kepri 2018 September.

Six weeks before Ironman Malaysia, I had a terrible sprain while running and had to stop peak training for two weeks. As my right ankle had chronic injuries since I was young, the ligaments were badly affected. Everyone nagged me not to attempt the race, but Sumit was my support, he said we will go and learn even if we don't finish.

On race morning, I was very anxious, my ankle was not hundred percent but maybe I could do this. I had a great swim and even managed to finish the bike course not too far from my goal time, I had six hours 45 mins to finish the run. At 13 km, my foot started hurting very badly. I was barely running, it was more like a slow walk drag of my foot, I was filled with doubt to continue or not.

At 22km, I sat down by the side of the road and had a chat with myself.

Mind: *If you quit it'll be a hattrick DNF, do you want to quit?*

Realistic me: *There is always another chance to come back.*

Mind: *What will your fellow trainees think?*

Realistic me: *I am racing for myself, not to prove to anyone else.*

Mind: *Will you be able to justify your efforts and your family's contribution?*

Realistic me: *I should not be so injured after the race that I become a burden on my family.*

I took a deep breath, closed my eyes and decided to quit at that point rather than try and finish the race and worsen my injury. It took a lot more mental courage to pull out than it did to sign up and train. I had promised Sumit I would come back whole and not broken. Next morning, I took the flight back home. I cried for many days though. I will go back another year soon, because I know I am persistent.

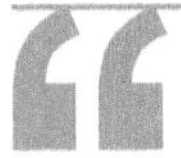 *"Stop comparing, race for yourself, is the principal learning in my athletics journey."* 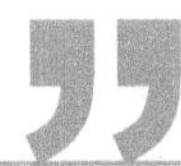

During my IM Malaysia training, I got carried away and started comparing myself to my fellow trainees. This made me push myself beyond my limits and capabilities, being in constant fatigue and prone to injuries. I have since logged out of strava and started training on my own under the supervision of my current friend-turned-coach Smita, who understands me and my problems. I took two years to recover from my injuries and slowly come back to my training.

Mom guilt is probably the biggest challenge I face. I used to train alone at ridiculous hours over the weekends just to make it back home in time for the kids' activities. As a mum the day doesn't end at the finish line of a race. I don't go back and rest, because I have to resume mom duties. In order to raise a happy family, the lady of the house has to be happy and filled with energy. So now I am resolved to making the boys more independent. I am not around most mornings, and they know I am training. My husband takes care of everything at that time.

I draw a lot of motivation from my family, my mother is a renowned rangoli artist, she has a Guinness record for the world's largest rangoli (2003), and my mother-in-law is a multi-talented woman, who, even at this age, finds new things to learn. My father-in-law, 76, is an avid walker, no matter the weather he won't miss his morning walks. My father started cycling during COVID-19 and raised funds for charity at 71 years of age. Both my kids and husband complete many races each year, including duathlons and fun runs.

I don't stop myself or restrict myself from trying new things; not even things that scare me. I am always making goals and going after them because I believe life is too short to spend complaining and regretting. If you want to do something, don't over think. That will happen. You will fail. So what? In life, it is not that you shouldn't fall, everyone is going to at some point, but it's important how fast you get up, dust off and move on.

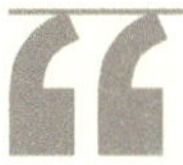

> *"Dance taught me passion and discipline, but triathlon taught me that I can apply these to any field."*

I have come a long way in my athletics life. I have met amazing people and made some very close friends, been part of encouraging groups (One Endurance Abu Dhabi, RockRunners, Rock The Naked Truth, Singapore Women's Triathlon, Indian Women's Triathlon club, Women's Cycling project, and many others) through my triathlon journey. I do wish to see more women, especially Indian Women in sports and triathlons.

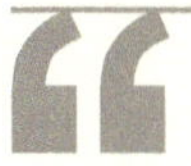

> *"I hope we can create a community that supports women, so that issues such as body shaming, sexual abuse, self-doubt do not hold them back from achieving their dreams. This is our responsibility for the next generation."*

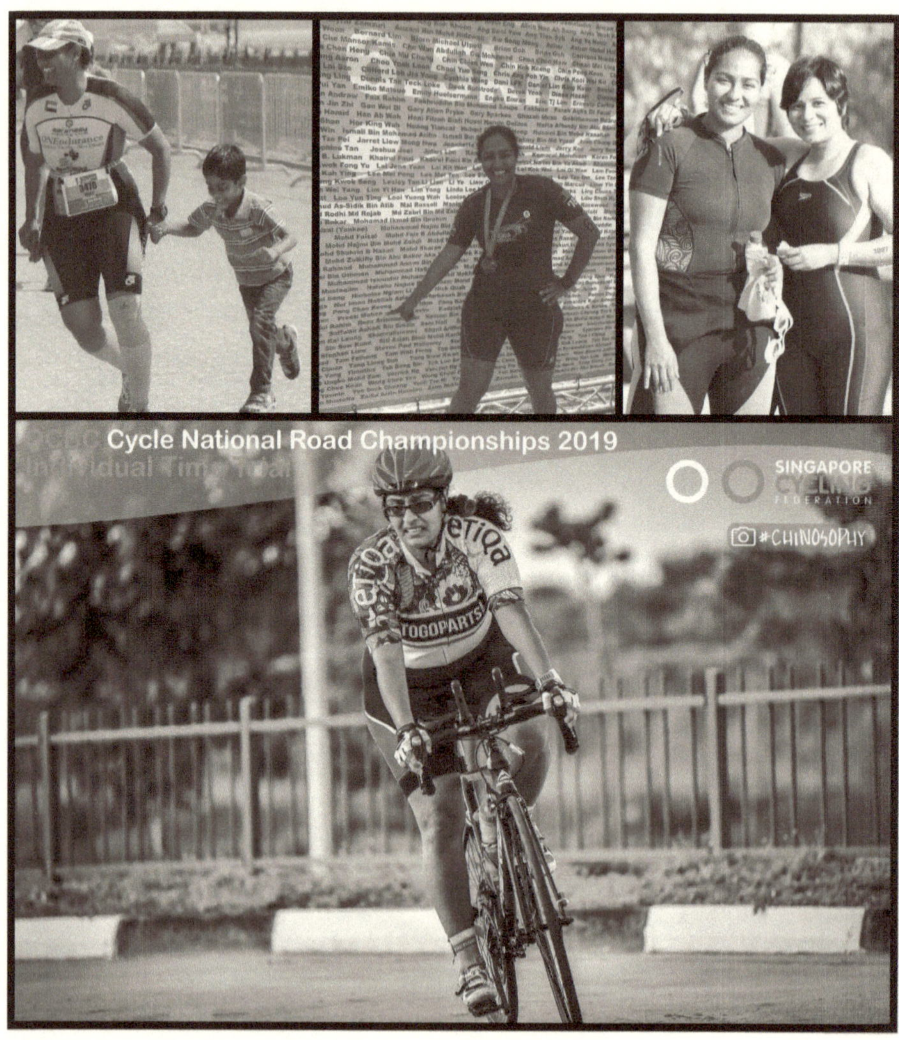
Cycle National Road Championships 2019
Individual Time Trial
SINGAPORE
CYCLING
FEDERATION
#CHINOSOPHY
etiqa
etiqa
TOGOPARTS

Strong is the New Beautiful

14

Dhunte Reh Jaoge – A Winner Who is Far from Social Media Fanfare

Dr. Uma Vinod, Ahmedabad

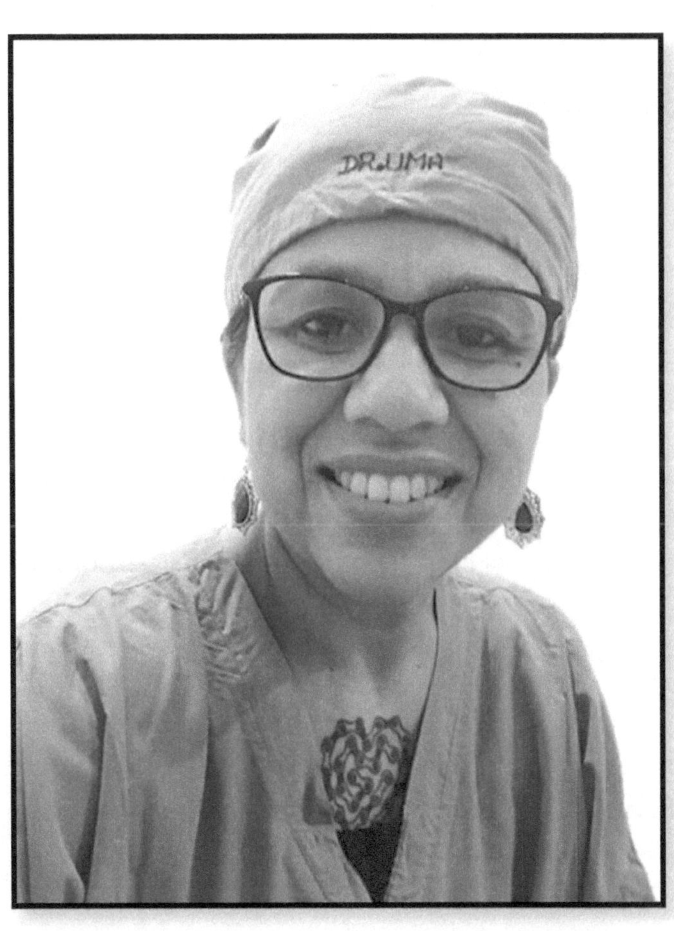

All that she needed was one visit to a racing arena and now, years later, she tells us how that moment changed everything for her. Meet 47-year-old Dr. Uma Vinod, an Ahmedabad-based Ophthalmologist and a mother of two boys, first rank holder of Gandhinagar Triathlon 2018 and winner of several cycle races.

"When I first saw the racing arena, zooming cycles, training jargons, and high energy at the event, I was almost hypnotized. I never imagined that such a world existed. I made up my mind that I'll be a part of all these high adrenaline events." I got married immediately after my MBBS and completed my Post Graduation in Ophthalmology. I was soon engrossed in all motherhood duties, work, and house chores—a typical story for most married women.

The Taste of Victory

In 2012, I participated in my first half marathon and finished in 3.45 hours. I was on cloud nine. In 2014, I witnessed a cyclothon in Ahmedabad. I was aghast to see the zooming cycles, the cheering crowd, and pumped up, high energy athletes. I was stunned by the entire event. I never imagined the existence of such a world, as if it was a parallel universe.

In the same year, I registered for a super sprint event. The main reason to register for the event was – Milind Soman (blushes). The race briefing was an eye-opener. I heard terms like wet-suit, cadence, cut-off timing, and several other jargons that were Greek to me. The trainers talked about cycle gear ratio and cleats while I came to participate in the race on my son's bicycle!

For the event, I got my first BSA "thin" tire bike assuming it'll make me go faster. Only thin tyres don't make you win a race-training and effort do. With all the learnings of the previous event, I got my first road bike and participated in a Duathlon in 2014. I stood first!

By now I was in deep love with cycling. I started participating in cycling races and winning too. I was utterly mesmerized by the sheer joy of zooming on the bike and winning as well. I was a hypothyroid patient until the age of 40, but then I decided to lead a healthy life and brought down my weight significantly.

Do It Because It Makes You Happy

In 2015, I went to Manali-Leh biking, and as it is known that the route is not for the lesser mortals. I was surely not the one. It was a life-changing experience for me. It was my Zen moment of putting all the elements of the body together and strengthening my mind.

I was gaining expertise in cycling, but was lagging behind in running. I started with proper training in 2017. Guided practice, along with a proper diet helps a lot in improving training performance. In 2018, I participated in the Triathlon in Gandhinagar. Due to fewer women participants, the organizers kept an open category for women 18–55. I stood first in the race!

I then registered myself for the Berlin Marathon in 2019. I was hesitant to go on my own, but my elder son persuaded me to travel. Technology and I don't have much of a friendship. To navigate the phone to find a way or even to use google translator is tough for me. But I did. Because it made me happy, very happy.

The Lesser Lady

I face the same set of questions each time,

➤ What fun do you get in killing yourself in training?

➤ You are always either running or cycling, do you even spend time with your family?

➤ Why are you going alone for your races, take your children along too?

➤ How will your family manage without you?

I'll miss cooking a great meal over the weekend, but I'll never miss my training, this gives me the title 'lesser lady.'

I mostly train alone and do not share that "ME" moment with anyone. It is my meditation. My alarm buzzes at 4 am and I go out for my run. It's dark at that hour so I can't go far; hence I run in loops at a stretch in front of my building. I have informed my guard that if I don't turn back within time or he hears my scream, then he should run to trace me.

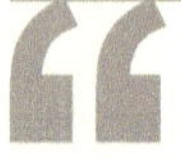

There will be questions, allegations, and stereotypes to face, but the choice is yours, either pay heed and remain in your cocoon or be a butterfly. What will you choose?

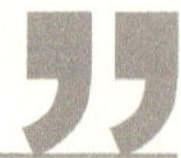

A Woman Among Boys

There are five male members in my family: husband, father-in-law, father, and two boys (18 and 15). I am a working female, and along with my training and work, the house responsibility doubles up. There were days when I could not prepare the meal, and my boys made their tiffin and went to school. In the growing years, my children understand cohesive existence. They also see that I have a liking towards sports gadgets than fancy clothes.

There was a point where I was fulfilling all my duties as a mother, wife, daughter, professional, but I wasn't doing anything for myself. It was a tough call to prioritize my liking over everything else. We live in a society where women are meant to be more focused on home, but I believe when you don't negotiate, you'll always be taken for granted. Today my elder one is studying in IIT Kharagpur and is in his college squash and running team. He is a swimmer as well. He says, "Mom, sports gave me recognition." He prefers a girlfriend who loves cycling! My younger one has already completed a triathlon and is looking forward to more.

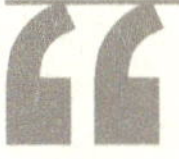

"Mothers are the first and most significant influencers, see that you prove this to yourself first."

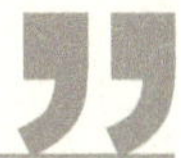

I aim to improve my race timings and keep winning as a mother, as an athlete, and emerge as a stronger version of myself.

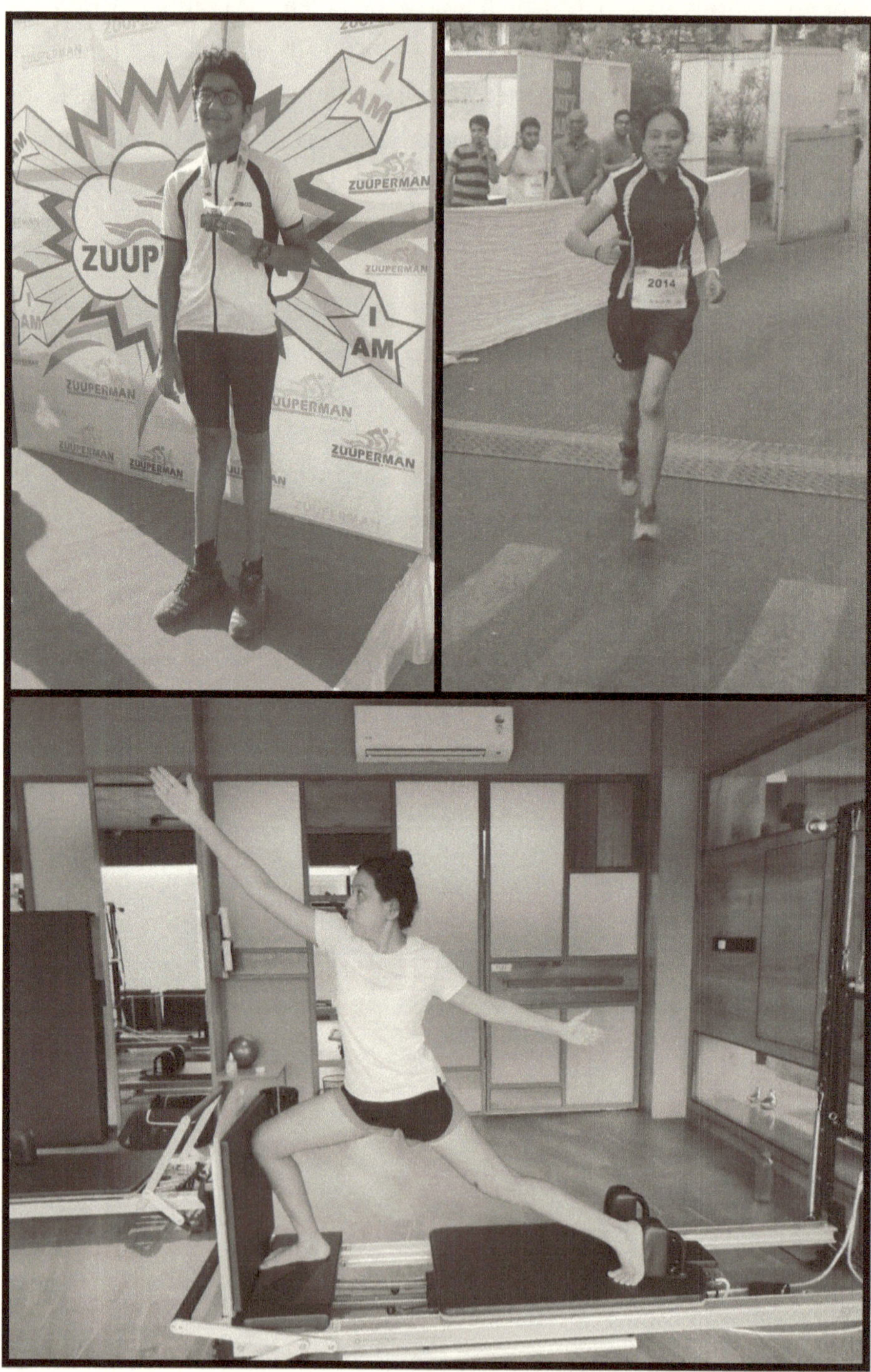

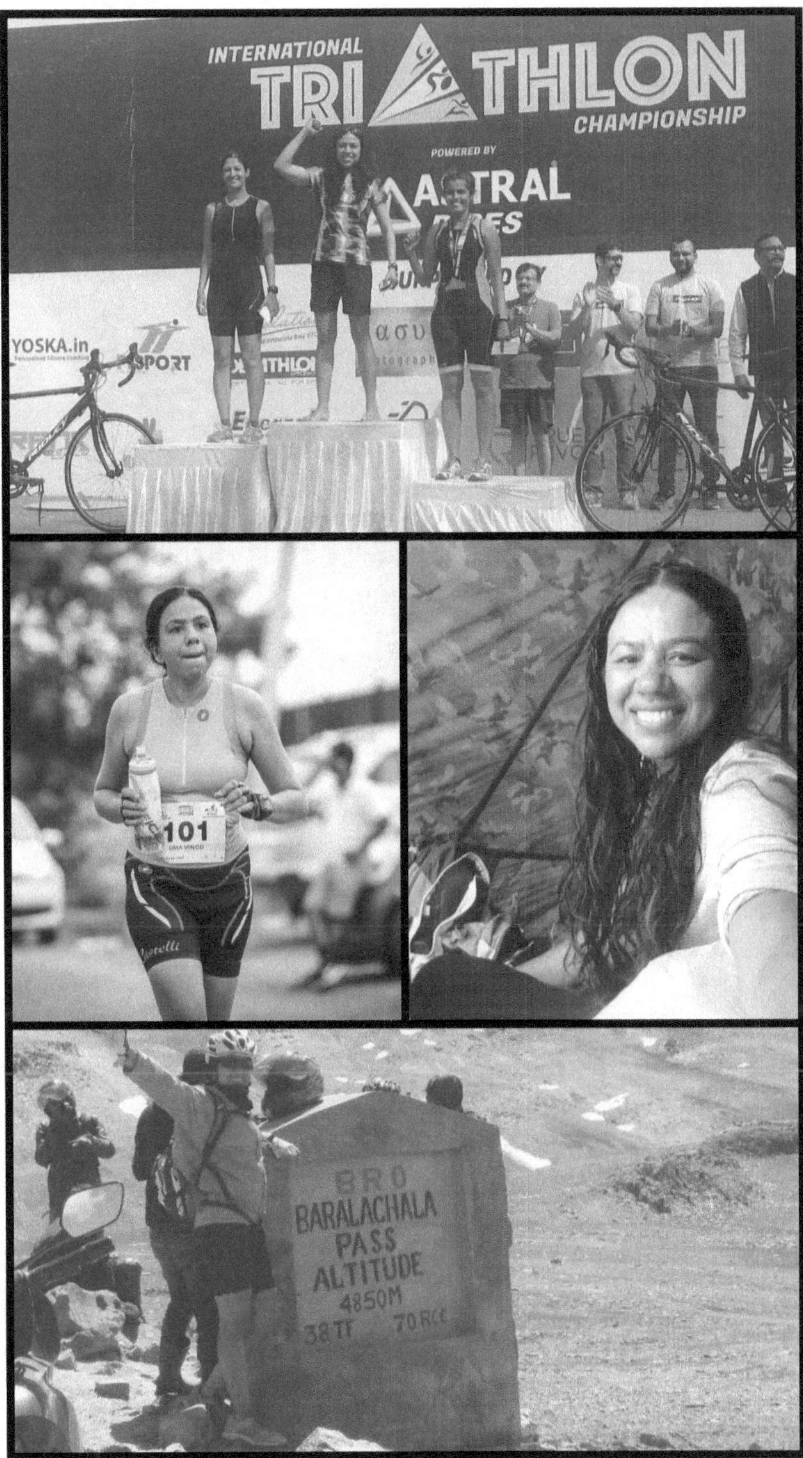
INTERNATIONAL
TRIATHLON
CHAMPIONSHIP
POWERED BY
ASTRAL
YOSKA.in
SPORT
101
BRO
BARALACHALA
PASS
ALTITUDE
4850M
38 TF   70 RCC

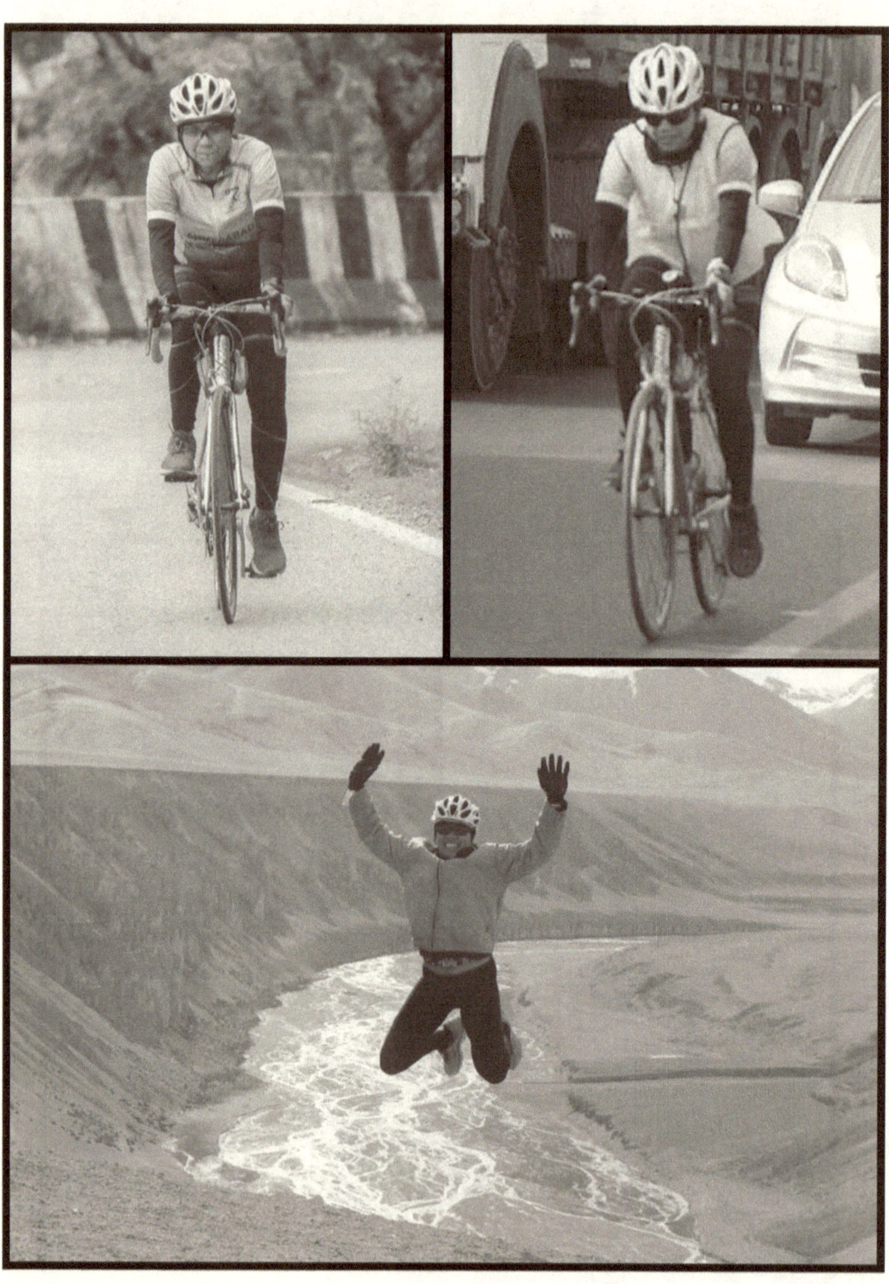

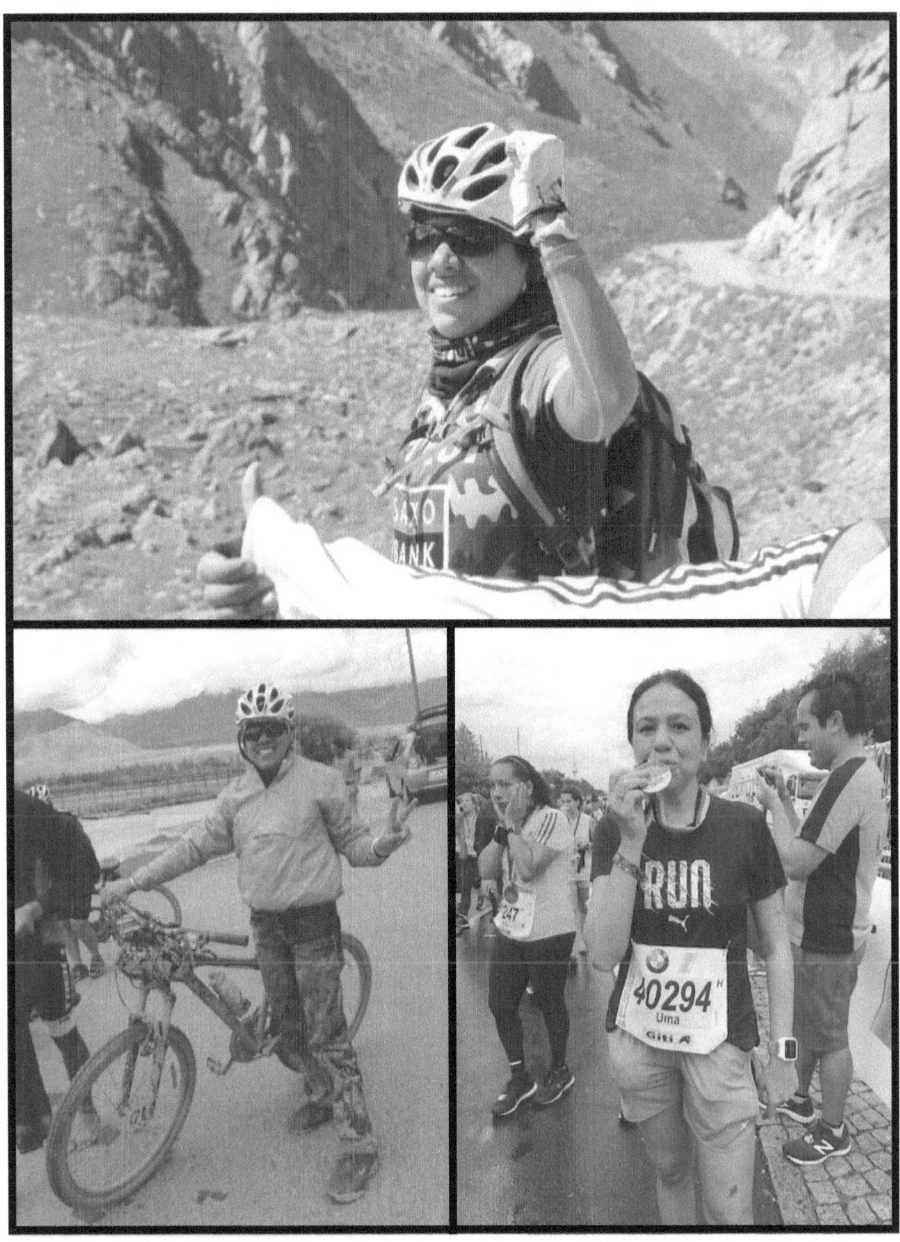

Races End, Running Doesn't

15

Sutli Bomb

Dr. Nandita Paranjape Joshi, Kolhapur

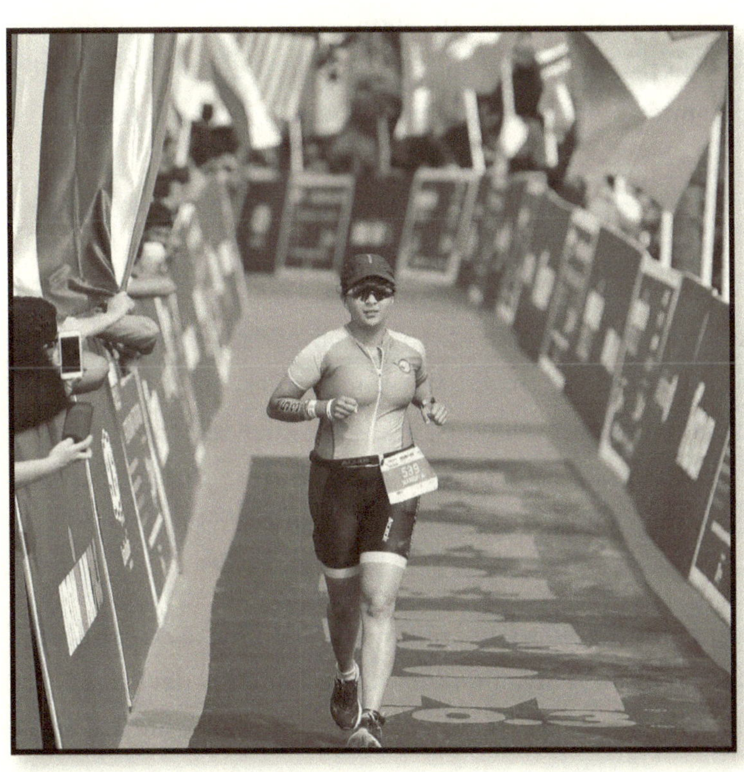

Once a patient of sciatica, backache, irritable bowel syndrome, permanent asthma, several health issues, poor lifestyle diseases; now an Ironman podium finisher. Kolhapur-based Dr. Nandita Paranjape Joshi is petite, small structured, 36 years old, mother of a five-year-old girl, gynecologist and infertility specialist and always hungry for more sport.

National Level Lawn Tennis Player

I had a beautiful childhood. There was a strict rule in my house that we siblings need to learn one art and one sport. I chose badminton but shifted to lawn tennis soon. I was pretty good at it (collars up). I represented Maharashtra thrice and played till nationals.

Back then, participation in tournaments was a simple affair without branded clothes and shoes. I am from Sangli, Maharashtra, a small laid-back town, and sport was all about strict training under my father's supervision. Our relationship during the training was not like father and daughter but as a coach and a trainee, hence there was no mercy.

Marriage, Children and Hectic Work Hours

Children always do the opposite of what their parents tell them, and I was no exception. I did my medicine even when my parents asked me not to. Both my parents are doctors, and they knew the long working hours in the profession. I completed my MBBS from Aurangabad and DGO too. I got married in 2010, and my daughter Nabha was born in 2015.

Nabha was eight months old when I resumed work. Due to stressful work hours, an infant at home, and an erratic work schedule, I developed a lot of lifestyle-related diseases. As the medical facility was easily accessible to me, I would do MRIs even for a minute symptom at the drop of a hat. I was in a persistent unhealthy phase. A childhood sports enthusiast was now under medicines and constant fatigue.

The Push

All thanks to my brother, who pushed me to get back on track. With a lot of reluctance, I joined lawn tennis again, my lost love. But lost love doesn't find existence in the present; hence I shifted to running. I could not even finish 400 meters in 35 minutes or so. I was huffing and panting all the time. My brother made me do a 10K in some event, which I finished in one hour and 40 minutes and slept off for two days. I cursed him with all my heart. Being a doctor myself, I sensed my alarming physical state. I had to take charge and so, I got into systematic training.

Races and Training

A structured training plan helped me get back to my earlier fit and good form quickly. I took great care of my diet, as well. In 2016 I did my first Kolhapur half marathon. Things were going fine until I met with an accident. I traveled to Spain for a conference where I had a terrible fall. MRI showed a ligament tear, and I was completely bedridden. All my hard work came to a standstill. I had to start from scratch now.

At this point, a friend who was not allowed to travel on her own for the event, registered me to the Belgaum Triathlon (sprint distance – 750 m swim, 20 km cycle, 5 km run). I had no idea about triathlons, I followed the race course, and to my surprise, stood third! I was utterly clueless. By now, I had started loving the entire endurance training and registered for the Kolhapur Triathlon, Olympic distance (1.5 km swim, 40 km cycle,10 km run), and stood second.

Then came the Goa Ironman, the first ever Ironman 70.3 (1.9 km swim, 90 km cycle, 21.1 km run) event in India, and I enthusiastically registered for it. I had never cycled 90 km before the race, and I seriously doubted my capability. Swimming is my strongest point as I have learned swimming in the river, but it was a tough course to tackle even then.

I was utterly exhausted in the last lap when I heard my husband and daughter cheering me, "Why are you walking? Run! You are in the second position. Go run to the finish line". I was pumped up immediately and finished second in my age category.

Training in a Small Town and Maharashtra Flood Hero

It is a challenging affair. I have to be careful on the route, the hour of the day, and the company during my training. I was advised to dress up like a boy to avoid eve-teasing. My training gear is either half or full-sleeves t-shirt and long tights. There are always a lot of questions from the society and even peer groups regarding my training.

At one point, I started doubting myself on my competency to manage my family, especially my child, and focusing more on the training. I shared my concern with my husband, and he assured me of going by what I think is right. As a woman, you have to prove your worth always, and it is pressuring.

During the Kolhapur floods in 2019, I promptly took charge to rescue the trapped people and saved 50 lives. My name flashed in all newspapers, and since then, there are no questions raised on my training or races.

Personal Growth

Endurance sport requires strict discipline, hard work, and a tough mind. It sharpens your thought process and decision-making ability. After strenuous training and long work hours, I used to get irritated and vent out my anger on Nabha. With a systematic approach towards training, I could manage my mood swings as well and developed self-awareness.

The field of Embryology and fertility requires precision, accuracy, empathy, attention to detail, emotional strength, and patience, and endurance training enabled me to acquire all these traits. I can tackle stereotyping with much grace and confidence. These things don't bother me anymore.

Does Hunger Continue?

Of course! It will. It has just begun. I aim to work for better stamina and much better timing in all my races. India lacks pro-athletes in international tournaments; I wish to represent India at the global platform.

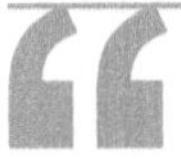

Be fearless and independent. Nabha wants me to be the next Lucy Charles, and I'll put all my efforts into being the best one from India.

Note to All Mothers

Extract one hour for yourself for your mental and physical well-being. Each one of us is unique and fighting our own battle. Comparison is the worst enemy for growth. Do not compare yourself to anyone, it spills a beautiful relationship called friendship.

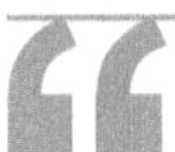

If you are happy, you'll keep your family happy.

P.S: Nandita is also a great cook and a sculptor. She's been making eco-friendly Ganpati idols for the last eight years at her home.

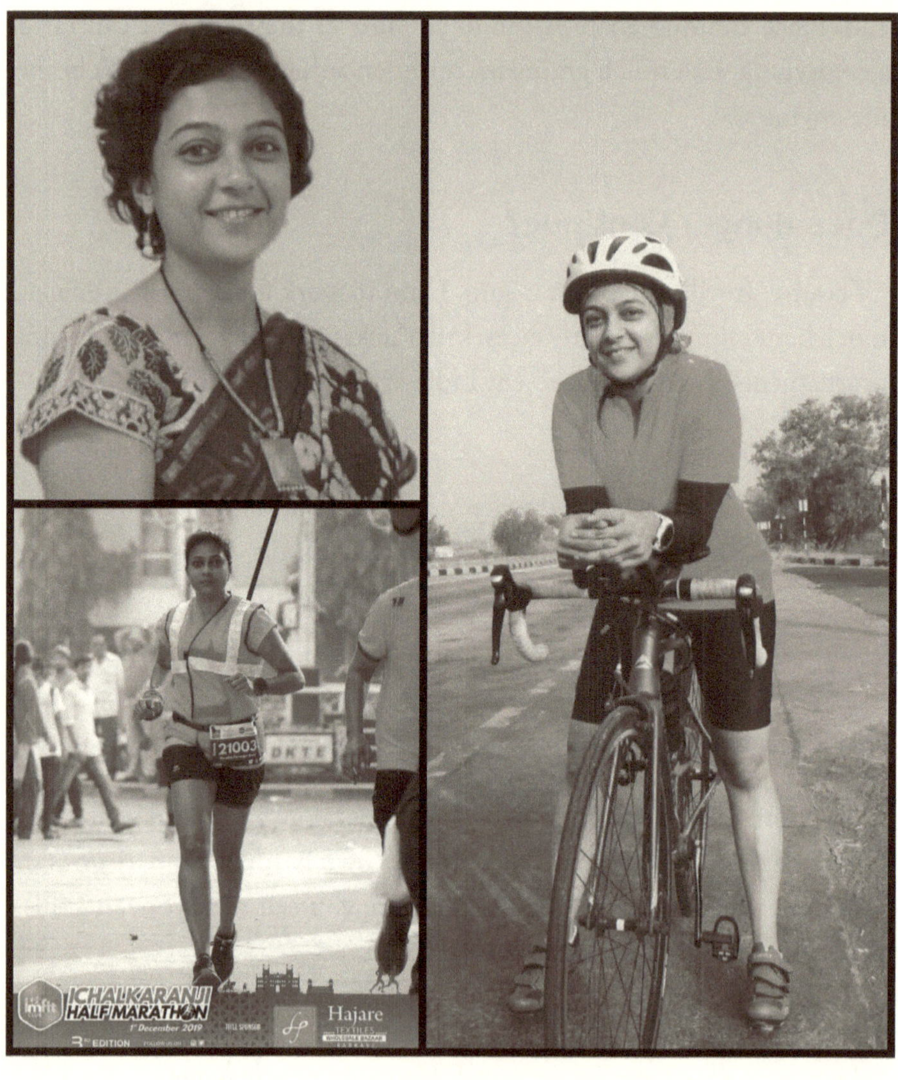
ICHALKARANJI
HALF MARATHON
1st December 2019
Hajare

Never Stop Dreaming 16

Snail-Paced Cyclist to a Podium Finisher

Ritu Kudal, Mumbai

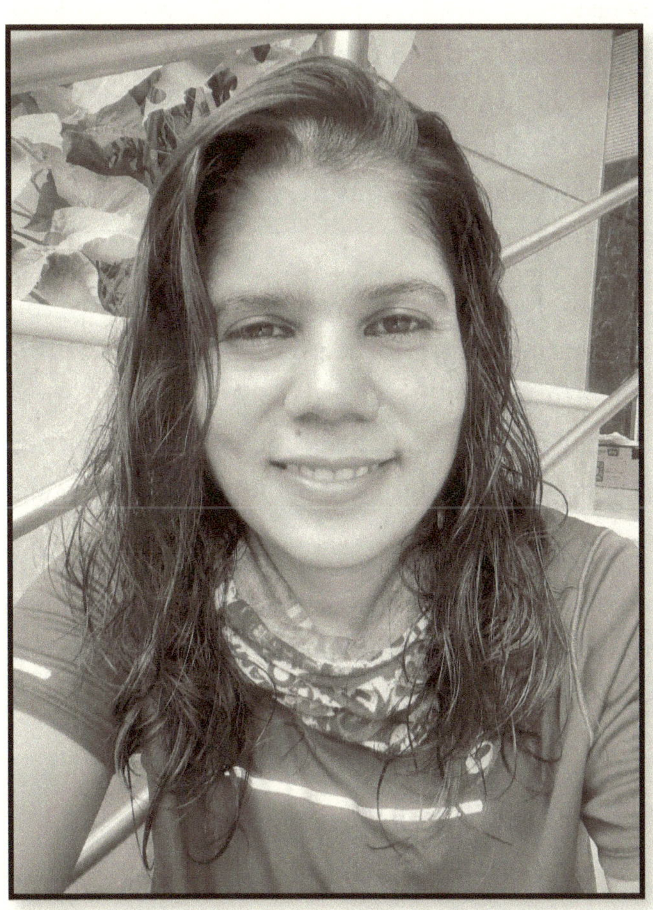

From a Marwari community of small town Udaipur(Rajasthan) to the city of big dreams Mumbai, from the pace of a snail to the only mother from Rajasthan finishing Ironman race, Mumbai-based, 41-year old Ritu Kudal, mother of two, has quite a few finisher medals in her kitty – Dubai 70.3 (1.9 km swim, 90 km bike, 21.1 run) 2020; Kolhapur 70.3, 2019 (Podium); Hyderabad 2018 (Olympic Distance – 1.5 km swim, 40 km cycling, and 10 km run), full marathon 2017, countless half marathons, 10 km and 25 km pacer; and she's determined to add more.

How It Started

I studied in Udaipur and was into sports from my childhood. Kho-Kho and running were my favorite sports. I have even played at the state level. I was selected for national level and had to travel to Nepal for the race; my mother was doubtful. Firstly, coming from a Marwari family, there was a stigma for girls to participate in sports, and secondly, pursuing sports was not a serious discussion. I was unsure, so I left where I started and continued to study further.

Soon I was married, but I am glad that my parents respected my opinion of finding an educated match for me. I came to Mumbai after marriage and continued to pursue my Chartered Accountant course. My husband, Tarun, being a CA himself, helped me in the completion of the course. I carried on with my duty as a dedicated housewife and managing children.

When my elder one was six months old, I started to learn swimming because that was an excuse to get out of my house. The oldest student in my swimming class was 60 years old.

There is no age to learn anything new
(First lesson)

It was during a Ganpati celebration, when I was sitting in a pandal holding my second child in my lap, when my elder daughter's gymnastics instructor uttered under his breath that I looked like Ganpati. I went home and looked at myself in the mirror, and he wasn't wrong. What had I done to myself? With a chubby body and bulging belly, I surely looked like Ganpati.

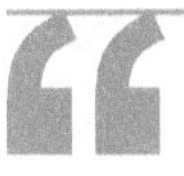
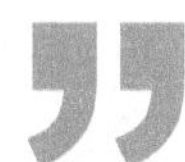

*Do not neglect yourself after childbirth. Your body needs a lot of attention. **(Second lesson)***

I developed hypothyroidism as well. I started walking and doing mild exercises until one-day, I met someone who had completed his half marathon. I was shocked by the distance he covered when I was struggling to walk even a 5K. When my younger one was six months old, I ran my first 10K Pinkathon race in 2013 and finished in one hour and two minutes.

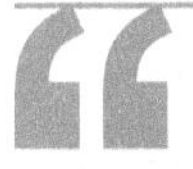

*It is always challenging to take the first step but dare to take it, and it'll make all the difference. **(Third lesson)***

There was no looking back then. I did the Goa marathon, Kundalika river; Marathon, Satara Hill run and after four years, in 2017, ran my first full marathon with systematic planning and training.

That Moment

My first Triathlon was Hyderabad 2018, Olympic distance. I chose to race here to test the waters, and surprisingly, I stood fourth in my age category. Next was Kolhapur 2019 70.3, and I faced open water swim (OWS). Ah! to face the fear of open water and then to swim through that distance was a tough task. I trained hard and was a podium finisher at the race.

Dubai 70.3 was announced by now, and after talking to Tarun, I registered. A race that I can never forget. My coach Viv Menon and swim coach Ashutosh left no stone unturned to turn me into a beast by grueling training plans. My day started early, and after preparing breakfast and packing my kid's tiffin boxes, I used to head for training. There were days when my body gave up, and my legs ached, but I had a massive target in front of me, and I didn't pause.

Before the race day, I packed my bike, learned how to mend the puncture, and made up my mind to travel alone. Yes, it was my first international trip on my own. It was a great accomplishment to get the visa stamped, issue a new SIM card, and manage everything on my own.

After the trial swim, I was down with a cough, cold and high fever. I panicked as my body was too weak to face a tough race ahead. On race day, my swim went well, but due to coughing I had gulped a lot of seawater, I started vomiting while cycling. My left side of the body was almost frozen, and I had severe pain. I was tense not because of my state, but what if something happens to me? I have children back home.

I was not going to accept a DNF (Did Not Finish), and I pushed myself hard to the finish line. The glimpse of the India flag at the finish line, the sense of victory and achievement took away all my pains, aches, fever, and anxiety. It was a moment of pride and triumph.

You have to put effort on your own to achieve the impossible. **(Fourth lesson)**

Gratitude

I am grateful to my parents, who ensured that I got proper education. I can't thank my coach Viv Menon, Ashutosh, enough, who pushed me hard and beyond my limits. Most importantly, I could have never done any of my races without Tarun. Whenever I step out for a competition, I always ask Tarun to put his hand on my head. It fills me with immense confidence and trust. That cheer from my kids, "Mom, you can do it!" kept ringing in my ears all through my racecourse.

Is the Hunger Over?

No, the hunger to chase the impossible will never get over. Once I was back from Dubai 70.3, I enrolled for the Goa swimathon for 5K. My coach asked me, "Are you ready to fail, Ritu?" I replied, "it's not about failing or timing, but I want to test myself." I am glad I took a plunge and finished the 5K swim.

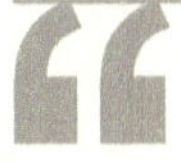

Dare to dream and have the courage to chase your dreams. What seems impossible now will become a reality soon.

My mantra

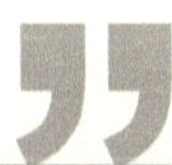

Getting married or having kids is no reason to stop you from achieving your dreams. Never stop learning, never stop dreaming, and be happy for yourself and on your own.

Dream. Believe. Chase. Achieve.

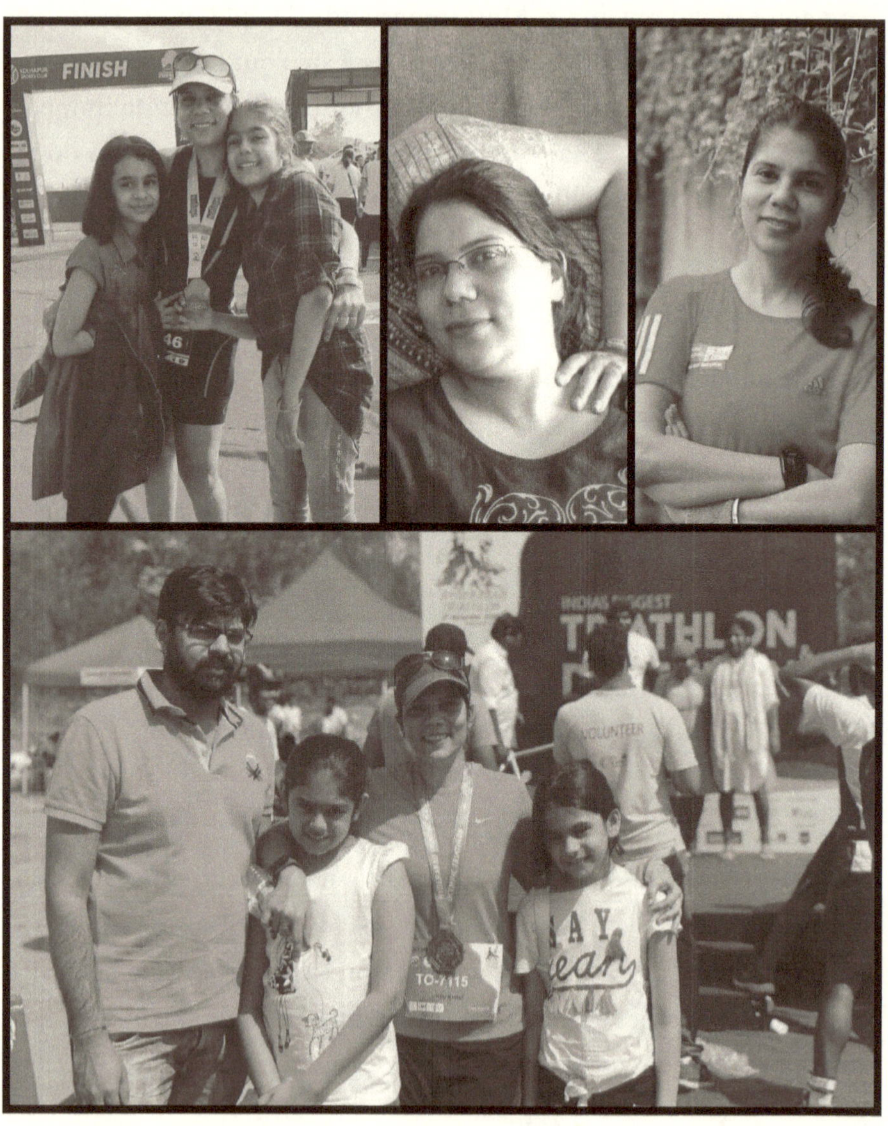

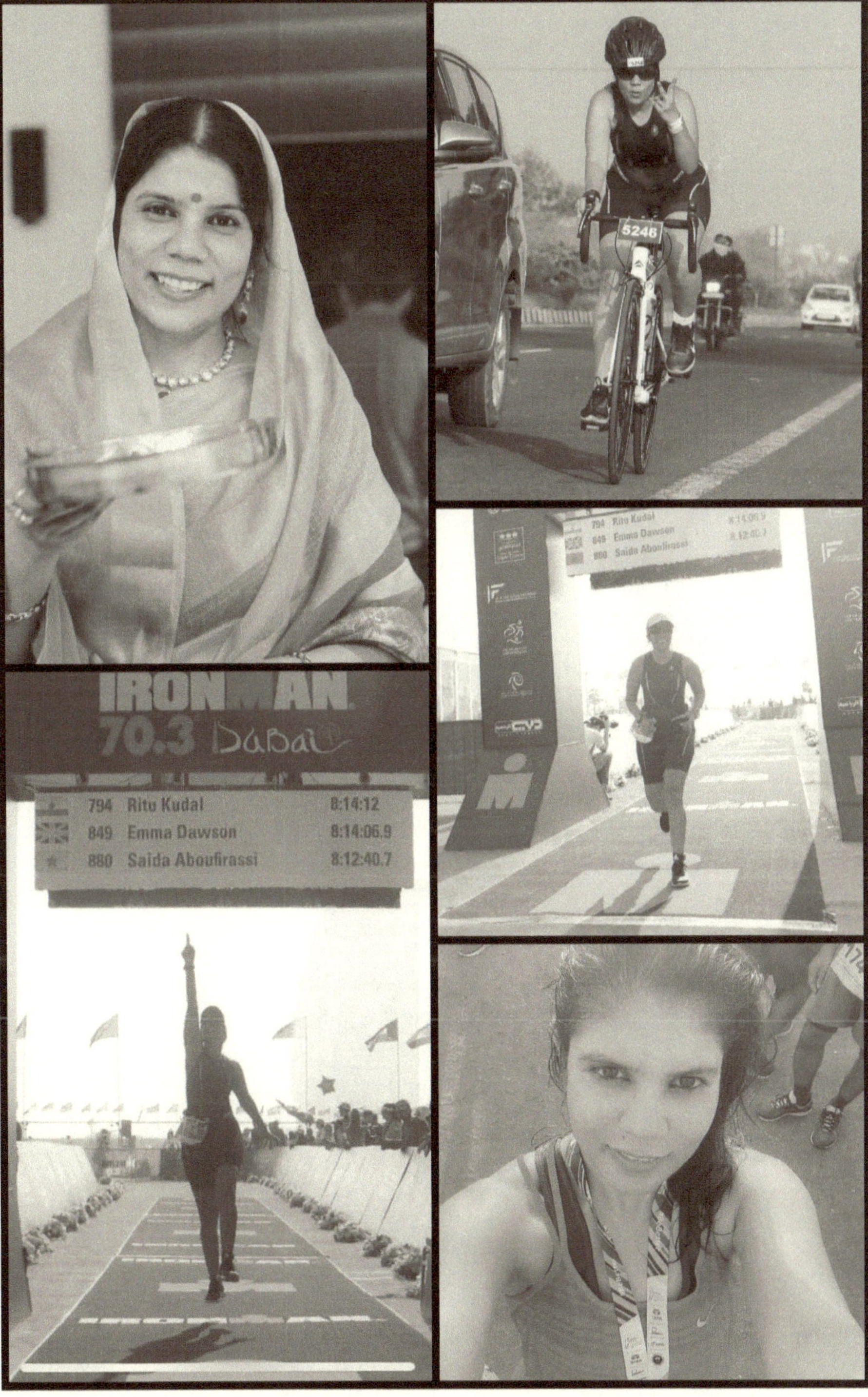
IRONMAN.
70.3 Dubai

794   Ritu Kudal   8:14:12
849   Emma Dawson   8:14:06.9
880   Saida Aboufirassi   8:12:40.7

5246

Every Race is a Journey

17

Enough is Also Not Enough

Vinolee, Chennai

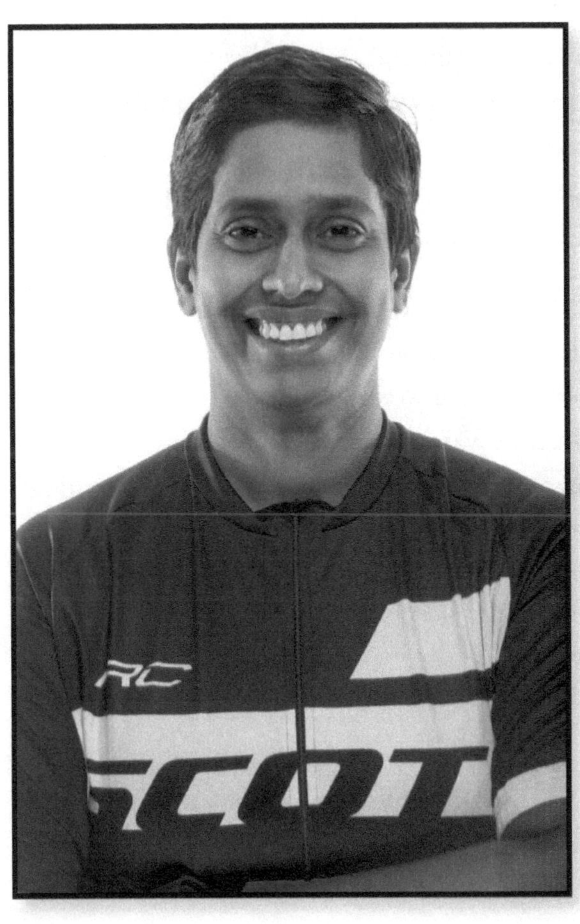

She was body shamed, abused on social media, had troubling weight and hormonal issues, but that was nothing compared to the support and confidence her family had in her. She's the first Indian woman to complete three IRONMAN 140.6, first woman from Tamil Nadu to complete Ironman 70.3 World Championship, France, 2019, first Indian woman to qualify twice in a row for Ironman 70.3 World Championships. Completed Ironman Barcelona 2017, Ironman Italy 2018 and Ironman Cairns, Australia 2019. From a college professor to a professional athlete, certified Ironman coach, here is 35-year old Vinolee Ramalingam's journey.

A Progressive Family

I come from a small town – Thanjavur. My father was always into athletics. In fact, he is also a national awardee. Unknowingly my training for Tri started at an early age. I had a fear of water, and any water body freaked me out. When I was quite young, my father just pushed me into the water. I had no choice but to swim.

I started representing the state and nationals in swimming when I was in Grade 3 and basketball, cycling and athletics and won accolades from Grade 8 onward. My brother was also an athlete. Whenever I had to choose between sports, athletics was my first choice. In 2000, I won my first national gold medal in athletics for 100m and 4x100m relay and one for basketball. I always dreamt of representing India at an international forum. The thought of holding the tri-color gave me goosebumps.

Work, Family and First Plunge

By 2008, I had finished my B.Tech and M.Tech. Due to my brother's sudden demise, I decided to continue with my studies and work while staying with my parents. I was an only child now, and my parents needed me.

I got married in 2010 and shifted to Chennai. After completing M.Tech., I had joined SRM Engineering College as an Assistant Professor. Now, life got tedious as travelling to and fro for work was long and tiring. Life revolved around bus-stops, college and home. I gained a lot of weight post-pregnancy.

My life was running on auto-pilot. I tried to go to the gym and follow a diet pattern, but everything seems impossible to follow due to irregular work hours. In 2016 I came across an event organized by the Chennai Trekking Club (CTC). My husband showed me a picture of the lake for the swim. Swimming has always been a strong sport, and I was mesmerized by the image. I was about to take a plunge after a gap of 15 years! This was my first Tri event. I struggled hard to keep myself fit, and worked hard on my negative areas and completed the event with a sense of accomplishment. The event consisted of a 1.9km swim, 90 km bike and 21km run.

With the 2016 Full Ironman on my mind, I decided to participate in the Hyderabad Ironman 3/4th race with no clue about the technical aspect of the race. This race has been the toughest. I could finish the pool swim of 2.3 km, the bike ride of 130 km easily, but the 32 km run was daunting. Seeing my struggle, the organizers advised me to quit. But the stubborn soul in me wouldn't quit. I reached the finish line. I could not complete the race within the cutoff time. With no practice and almost negligible body strength, I was still the only woman to finish the race.

In 2017, I was the only woman participant to finish the 15KM Swimmathon conducted by CTC Chennai (2017). It was time to take a complete U-turn now.

Going After My Life Goals

There was a buzz about Triathlon. The curious cat in me gathered more information and found it interesting. Taking into consideration my gap from athletics and my weight gain, I decided to participate in the half iron category – swim 1.2 mile (1900 meters), bike for 56 miles (90 km), and run for 13.1 miles (21 km). Swimming came easy to me but due to a lack of stamina, I was lagging in running. I didn't even have a cycle, and wearing a helmet was something new to me.

I made training plans independently and with much reluctance, yet with a firm mind, I finished Ironman 140.6 organized by CTC Chennai in 2016 and 2017. I led the swimming course, but I missed being a podium finisher as running is my weakest sport. For a moment, I was disheartened. I've always believed that the podium is not life, but it's a challenge to myself – to chase my life goals. I worked hard for a year, managing strict working hours and also working on my body. In 2018, I stood a winner at the International Triathlon Championship in 70.3 Ironman distance in Gujarat.

Unstoppable Me

I was progressing slowly but reasonably well. Slowly and steadily, I started to learn more about the races and the terms. Bodyweight and poor running form were still an issue for me. Although the working hours were strenuous, my focus was firm.

Barcelona Ironman 140.6, 2017

I got to know about a triathlon race in Barcelona, and it attracted my attention. I wasn't sure how to register for an international event. Google came to my rescue. I noted down everything like a sincere student, prepared an Excel sheet and jotted all the pointers – the course, elevation, cut off timing, the country's temperature, and other factors.

The next hurdle was to take necessary permission from the college and plan the trip's budget.

My friend Ashwin briefed me about the racecourse, and I was petrified to know about the elevation. I had just four months to prepare, and I was not ready to fail. Seeing my dilemma, he suggested that I keep this race as a target and chase it with all my might. I did so.

Four months went in a jiffy, and I was all set for my first ever international race. We reached Barcelona three days before the event. It was our first trip outside India, and we all were anxious. Once I assembled the bike, I went for a trial and faced two punctures. Although I knew how to mend the puncture, it took me 30 mins. I mentally prepared myself to hurry up because I'd lose time in the race in case of such a mishap.

On the bib collection day, the officials informed us that wetsuit was a compulsory requirement for the race. I wasn't carrying one and so, rented one for the race. The swim trial was challenging in a wetsuit. I have a heavy chest, and the wetsuit was suffocating. My limbs felt stuck, and I was breathless. Standing at the shore, I was almost in tears, even though swimming was my strongest sport, I felt choked. I closed my eyes, meditated for a while, and remembered what all I had gone through for this race. I found my heart beat coming back to normal.

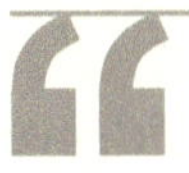

"If your mind is free you can perform way better than your practice."

I completed the swim course in one hour and 20 minutes, and gracefully finished the race in 14 hours and 53 minutes.

Italy 2018

Once back from the race, I was back to college and house chores. There was hardly any time left for the training. It was getting difficult to focus on work, home and training in parallel. My husband understood my confused state of mind and suggested that I leave the job and focus only on training. I was doubtful. Triathlon is an expensive sport, and if I left my job, our household income would cut to half. I mulled over it and finally took the tough decision, going by my husband's belief and confidence. I left my job.

Now, my single-point focus was Ironman, Italy. I learnt that the course was tough with difficult hill climbs. Hence, I trained hard with hill reps. We used to drive 300 km away from my house, my son and husband would be in the car while I practiced the climbs. I laid emphasis on my running form as well.

We reached Italy a week before the race. Upon arrival, we lost our baggage. We only had our backpack left with us. We somehow managed to reach our hotel. Being on a stringent budget, it was tough to have a proper diet.

I received my bike after two days. Due to inadequate hydration, I got cramps while swimming. Cycling was not easy either, as I had two falls. Running anyhow being the most challenging vertical in triathlons, was tough to tackle. I was dehydrated. I had no idea about energy drinks or gels. I somehow managed to finish the race in 15.27 hours.

I was utterly disappointed with myself. I thought about the confidence my husband had in me. How much my young son had contributed to my training by being patient. And, here I was putting up an abysmal performance. That race taught me many life lessons. At this point, I realized that although it is essential to be fast in a race, it is equally important to build up endurance strength and take care of all other aspects for a more robust finish.

Colombo, SriLanka, 2019

With prior experience, I was reasonably prepared for this one. My weight was still an issue, but I now focused on my strong points. I successfully finished the race in six hours and 42 minutes. Although I stood sixth in my age category, I qualified for the Ironman70.3 World Championship, Nice, France. I completed the championship in under eight hours. I am grateful for all the forces that backed me with immense energy for the world championship qualifier.

Cairns, 2019

Cairns is known for a challenging route, extreme weather conditions and a rough sea. Race officials also mentioned that we might have crocodiles and sharks as our co-swimmers. It was creepy. We reached the race site a week prior. It was important for me to get acclimatized. Due to the rough sea, I wasn't allowed a trial swim. I would go to the beach each day and stand there, gazing at the sea. The sight gave me jitters. For the first time, I started doubting myself. The confusion was visible on my face.

Rakesh comforted me. He told me not to worry about the DNF but to take learnings at every step. I had always stood tall with his confidence, and when the swim trial opened, although jittery, I set my foot and stretched my arms in the sea. On the race day, the sea was at its worst behavior. With my eyes closed, I visualized my son and husband at the finish line, and it was enough for me to plunge into those waves. I finished the swim in one hour and 24 minutes. The first lap of cycling was smooth, but then the headwinds came thrashing into my face. It was a challenging task to battle those winds. I kept chanting a mantra, "Do or die, and I am surely not dying." I touched the finish line in 15 hours and 23 minutes.

Ironman 70.3 World Championships, Nice 2019

I was eager to reach France. We reached there five days before the event. This time, it was hassle free with our baggage intact. Nice has the toughest bike route with 40 km climb in a 90 km cycling route.

I wanted to try it out at least once before the race. The day after we landed, I headed for a practice ride. I ended up doing 70% of the route as I was lost halfway, with my mobile draining out. I was out on the road the whole day and somehow managed to reach the hotel. But this helped me in successfully completing the event.

It was a struggle in every race to reach the finish line but for this race, I touched the red carpet with a wide smile. I got the perfect finishing photo too and completed the entire course in seven hours and 50 mins. Races, training, routine and discipline became my second name.

Upon completing Ironman 70.3 Shanghai, China, I got qualified for the Ironman 70.3 World championship, Taupo, New Zealand, 2020, making me the only woman from India to be prepared for the 70.3 world championship twice in a row. I am waiting for the event to give in my best.

Training in a Pandemic

With the world coming to a halt, I had time to attend to my injuries and aching muscles. I spent a lot of my time at my native and focused on strength training. Rice bags became my weights and my father's old cycle my cycle trainer. Once back to Chennai, I started going out for cycling and running. This time helped me to work on my weak points and focus on my strength. I was also able to devote more time to my family as well.

What Made Me Who I Am

Small-Town Girl

I was born and brought up in a tiny town. My father never differentiated between my brother and me. I grew up listening to his race stories and what it takes to build an athlete. His achievement taught me two major traits, discipline and sincerity. From a very young age, my father showed much confidence in me and allowed me to make my own decisions. He made me travel independently in local transport for an event when I was just 11 years old. I came back home with a medal dangling around my neck. I have never let him down since.

The Only Girl in a Boys' World

I have always been the only girl in most of the competitions. Boys have more physical ability than girls, and competing with them made me push beyond my limits. I always won all athletic events, surpassing boys. My school supported me a lot and encouraged me to participate in all competitions without pressuring me to study. I wish that India should have such an education system where every child is encouraged to participate in sports and grades become secondary.

Leaving My Job

Leaving my job was a tough call. I lost my financial independence; our household income reduced, and managing training expenses was challenging. While discussing my confusion with my father and husband, they told me, "Vinolee, you are qualified enough to get back to work whenever you wish to, but it is equally important to follow your passion and accomplish your dreams. Do it now." For one of my races, I raised money through a fundraiser. I don't have any help at home as I do all chores on my own. There are lots of ways and means by which we save money for my events.

My Partner, My Strongest Pillar of Support

I married Rakesh in 2010. He always stands by me in all my choices, anxiety, fears, doubts, accomplishments, failures. I can lean on him whenever I need strong support. He has seen me cry, comforted me and held me tight when I was about to fall. At every finish line, my son and he are my loudest cheerleaders. That one loud cheer from my son, "Momma, you can do it" is enough for me to reach the finish line with a grin. They accept me the way I am. Rakesh is my critic too. He prepares my race performance report and then discusses where I went wrong. My Family is my mentor, coach, teacher, supporter and cheerleaders.

Mummy Guilt

Yes, I do feel guilty of leaving my job, pulling in my family at 3 am for training as my husband drives and son sleeps in the rear seat and unable to dedicate time to my son during training days. I have shared my guilt story with my family, and all they have to say is – "Be a winner, we are there with you, always."

Weight Issues and Body Shaming

Thyroid, hormonal imbalance and lots of accumulated body weight post-pregnancy made running tough for me. After Barcelona, I took structured training and was able to cut off both weight and running time. I reduced fat, but my thighs and breasts were heavy. The doctors advised me to undergo some hormonal surgery, but I refused.

After my accomplishments, Scott sponsored a bike, and Unived sports, nutrition. I posted a few pictures on social media with the bike, and I got some hideous comments on the post – my body, weight and capability were questioned. My husband was upset when he saw the comments; this disturbed me. I filed a complaint against the abusers. I wanted to clarify that no one is allowed to comment on any woman about her body type or skin color.

I made the message loud and clear – don't do this to any woman. Social media is a great tool to inspire people. It is equally important to understand that social media fame is short-lived. My postings tell my story of strength and determination. The body that we are dwelling in is short-lived, but the experiences that we have in our heart is immortal.

Periods and Training

I have a tough periodic cycle. I take adequate rest during my period as any workout leaves me with a high fever. Whenever I feel fatigued or tired, I immediately pause my activities and allow my body to take rest and recover adequately.

My Triathlon Journey

Competition exists, and it should because it helps you attain what your mind cannot. Competition for me is breaking my record, getting better in each way, finishing with courage, and never letting any finish hit my ego. After specific episodes, I have also ensured that I'd never compare myself with anyone. The only comparison is my performance, and it helps me in moving forward. I always believe that your dream is exclusive, so keep the dream alive in your heart and chase it.

Getting motivated is essential, but your identity is you. My triathlon journey has taught me that family comes first. I shall always remain indebted to them for the effort, dedication and sacrifice made for me to achieve my goals. Each race is a journey, and the medal tells the story of the force behind me.

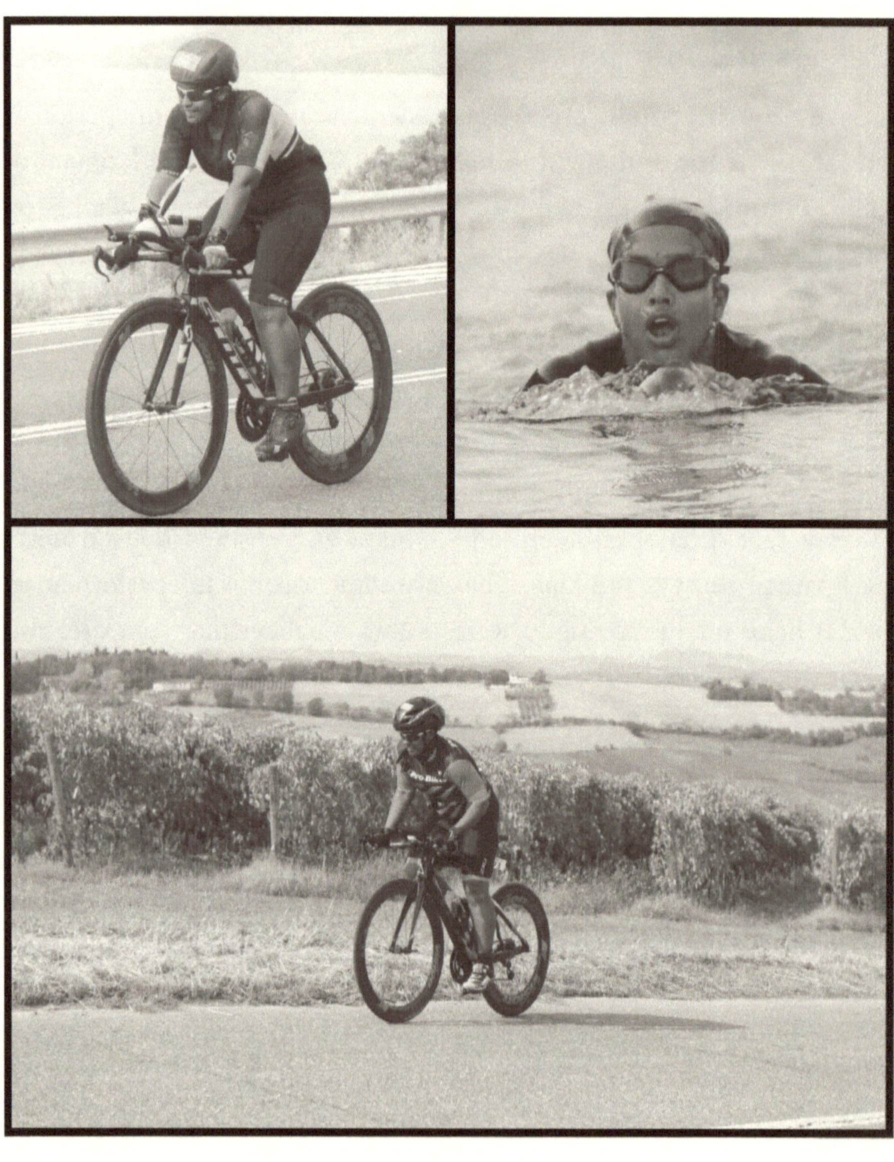

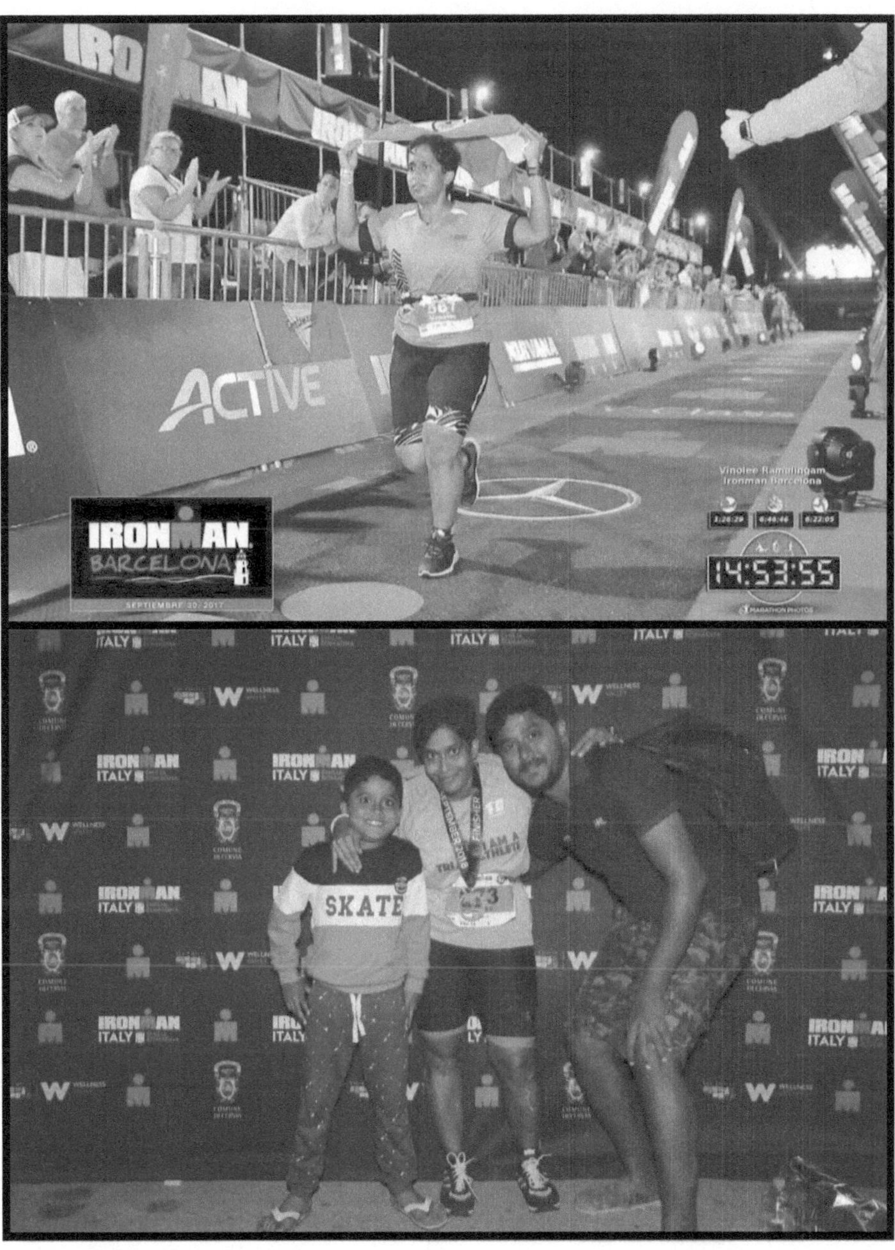

Tough is Not Your Body But Mind   18

Bundle of Energy

Disha Shrivastava, Mumbai

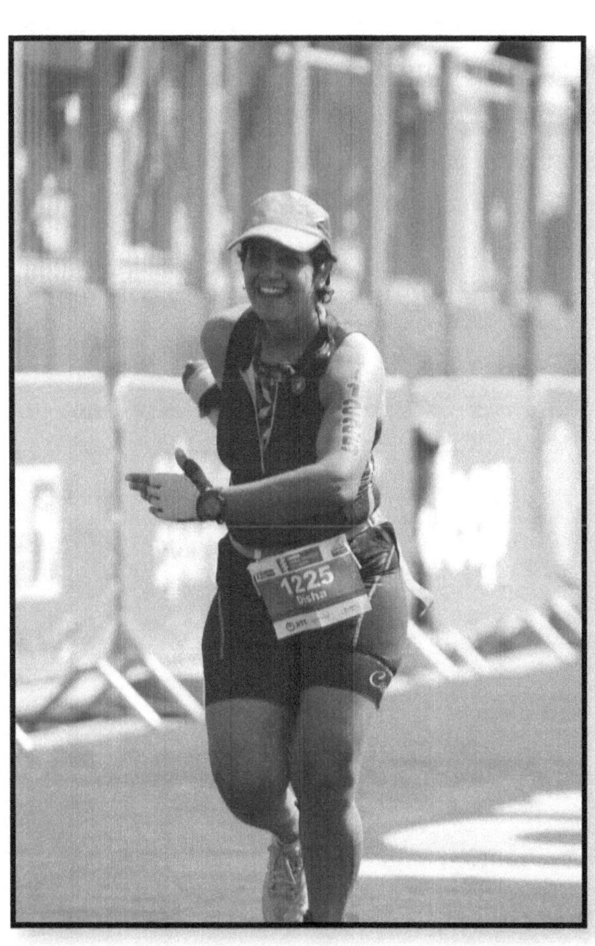

A working mom, entrepreneur, enthusiastic athlete, passionate runner, an explorer on a bicycle, dance lover, insanely emotional, always high on life, with numerous half marathons in her kitty, a woman with infectious energy, endurance is her second name. Finisher of Abu Dhabi ITU, here is 41-year-old, mother of two boys and a pet dog, Mumbai-based Disha.

Dance, Debates and Extracurricular

To start with, I spent most of my childhood in BHEL, Jhansi. I had a liberal upbringing, moreover, an upper hand in all the sibling fights as I was the youngest one with two elder brothers. I was my Papa's pet. We were a cohesive family. My father involved me in all kinds of chores, like mending electrical connections, changing cylinders, car maintenance and even made me travel on my own in local public transport. I thank him for making me ferociously independent. During my academic days, I was into dance, debate and elocution. I have won several national level accolades in debate competitions. It was an honour to be awarded as the Best Speaker, Youth Congress in Republic Day felicitation, New Delhi, 1999.

I used to participate in 100-meter track races, high jump and shot put at my school sports day, but that was it in sports. I was keen to pursue arts and dramatics and was also qualified for NSD, but as science is a more respectable subject than arts, I graduated in science. With no career guidance, no orientation and no aim, I was clueless about my career. I completed my MBA in marketing, got a placement and shifted to Mumbai.

Postpartum Downside

My aim in life was to get married and have children. I am a huge Bollywood fan, and I visualized my life as a Karan Johar movie. People often tell me that I live in a dream world, and I wouldn't deny it. I find magic and fantasy in everything around me.

I got married in 2004, and subsequently, Sid, my elder son, was born in 2006. Soon, we shifted to Gurgaon. I was a full-time mother now. Being a young mom at 26, I was overwhelmed by motherhood and hormonal changes causing havoc. As Sid started completing his milestones, I generally turned out to be anxious, irritated and short-tempered all the time. I was always screaming, throwing things and at times, even hitting Sid.

Sid was absorbing all the negative vibes, and it was showing in his behavior. There were constant complaints from the playschool and neighbors. As a consequence, I would scold my two-year-old baby rather than paying heed to my behavior.

In 2008, we shifted to Bangalore, and Abhi, my younger one was born in 2009. I was decently behaved this time but still not up to the mark. In 2011, when we shifted back to Mumbai, things hit rock bottom. I realized the severity of my situation when I thought of jumping off my 14th-floor balcony along with my two children.

I am still grateful that I didn't.

I have a vivid memory of the episode, and I am glad I do. Since then, I have Acrophobia.

Holding Myself Uptight

The reins of my battered state needed to be held together and tamed. With no help around and no one to talk to, share or understand, I was the sole warrior in this battle. I went back to my first love – dancing.

Being a full-time mom was challenging, and stepping out of the house wasn't easy. I started taking my children along with me for the dance sessions. Next, I came across a running group in my compound. Within no time, I joined it and started getting out in the wee hours for runs. I was a huge mommy, weighing 79 kgs, and running wasn't easy. I remember the days when even a 100-meter brisk walk was difficult. I did not give up and kept trying, one step after another.

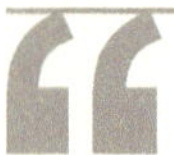

"I've carried a child within my body. I've slept with them on my chest. I've kissed toes and wiped away tears. I've been vomited on, peed on, and spent sleepless nights cradling my child. But I wouldn't have it any other way. My body isn't magazine perfect but when I look in the mirror, I see a mama. And there is no greater honor, love or blessing."

I did my first half marathon (Standard Chartered Mumbai Marathon) in 2015 and finished in three hours and 18 minutes. I distinctly remember how I dragged myself to the train station and got back home. I was exhausted, injured and drained. Although the finish line is ecstatic, I was utterly disappointed with my performance. I continued to run but also started with weight training in the gym.

"Recognizing that the power of will is the Supreme Court over all other departments of my mind, I will exercise it daily, when I need the urge to action for any purpose; and I will form HABIT designed to bring the power of my will into action at least once daily"

Bruce Lee

Moving Ahead Never to Look Back Again

A breakthrough came in June 2015. I was selected as the only female participant alongside 11 male participants across India by Times Passion Trail for a mountain biking event across Bhutan. With an overdose of confidence in my kitty and zero stamina, I was all set for the ten-day trail.

I was always the last one on the trail and could not even finish the desired distance each day. This trip to Bhutan made me realize many things:

➤ It is wonderful to pursue what you like.

➤ It is mandatory to realize your potential.

➤ Motherhood is endearing but do not soak yourself in the process.

➤ The female body is very complex and needs lots of care and attention post-pregnancy; so, show adequate love and care to your body.

Once, back from the trip, I was on fire. I started cycling regularly; long distances, too.

2015 – First trip across Rajasthan on my foldie

2016 – GoechaLa Trek, Sikkim

2016 – Met with an accident and got a metal rod in my hand

2017 – India Gate to Wagah Border, a ride for mental health awareness

2017 – Hampta Pass Trek

2017 – Another accident, but thankfully no broken bones

2018 – Tour de Chhattisgarh

2018 – Annapurna Circuit with Sid

2018 – Ride across Europe

2018 – First Triathlon

2019 – Ride across Vietnam

2019 – Successful second Triathlon

2020 – Built my core and endurance

I kept building myself every moment. I worked hard on moving out of my mommy guilt, stereotypes and expectations set on me. I focused my energy on endurance training. My world was all about work, training, kids and most importantly, self.

As the famous dictum goes, "Your vibe attracts your tribe", I increasingly started getting attracted to enthusiastic sportspeople and clubs.

Entry Into the World of Tri

It started over coffee when I met Mehul one evening in May 2018. He suggested I enroll in the Kolhapur Triathlon. I looked at him aghast, wondering – REALLY?! He discussed the race casually. Of course, he was casual because he's a pro at all sports and an Ironman. But what about me? Good at none.

I thought of giving it a shot. I had to streamline my workout and get into further strict discipline, so I needed a coach, and unanimously it was Viv. His weekly training plans left me breathless, exhausted, with sore muscles, but extremely satisfied.

I followed a proper diet and adhered to my training routine; my gym instructor, Sagar, framed my sessions as per my training plan; I tweaked and adjusted the plan with my travel and my kids' schedules.

I had to time my training and home, kids, work, travel and all of it, equally demanding. It's tough to burn the ass on the cycle trainer and simultaneously teach geography to your kid for a test.

DNF and the Finish

November 2018, I was all set for my first triathlon – excited, anxious, nervous, running cold, parched throat, dizzy, etc. On the day of the open lake practice swim, it took me several minutes to take the plunge. Finally, I managed but swam along the support rope for a short distance. I tried several times but could not achieve the full length.

I suffer from Acrophobia (fear of heights) and during this process realized that I also suffer from Thalassophobia (fear of water, dark, uncertainty). I studied a lot about it, talked to therapists, read several self-help books, but nothing helped.

I had a DNF (Did Not Finish) at the Kolhapur Triathlon. I could not swim even 100 meters in the race. I had to take this phobia in my stride, and **I always believe that nothing is more powerful than the human mind.**

Sheetal came to me as a guiding angel and introduced me to Nimesh, a swimming coach who took groups for sea swims. I had an anchor now.

I distinctly remember when I went for the open water swim for the first time — the night before, I was crying, praying, and meditating endlessly. At 4 am, I took a deep breath and drove to Uran, a two-hour drive from my place. The sea was low, and I swam only until where my feet touched the ground.

The second attempt was better than the first one. In the third attempt, I was confident, where I jumped into the middle of the sea from the boat and swam till the shore. The sea was high and the waves pushed me, but I managed to swim.

I still battle OWS (open water swim) fear as somehow the past experience is yet not out of the system but I am fighting and shall continue to do so.

Abu Dhabi Triathlon, March 2019

On the trial swim day, I took a while to jump in the water, but then I finally tried the sprint distance of 750 meters and was happy and confident to swim through the whole length the next day.

I was back at the hotel with a terrible throat ache, and by evening I was down with high fever. I rinsed and gargled with whatever medicines I had. Even sipping water was painful. I was terrified about the race now.

On the race day, I had a poor swim, but I was determined to finish the full distance and not give up. Once out of sea, I ran to T1 to get the bike and realized that I had not kept my glasses (I use high power glasses for the swim and run), I wore my swimming goggles instead. Finished the bike lap and rushed for the run. The sun was raging by now, and I held my chin up and jogged–ran–jogged and finally sprinted in the last lap cheering to myself, the way I do for Sid for his runs. I remember cheering loudly, **"*Sid, ho gaya* darling, almost done. Just 500 meters left, we will not give up. Run darling run. Mamma is right here with you."**

Once I touched the finish line, I sat down and cried my heart out, elated, that I just did not finish the race but I didn't give up even when my body did. And I never will.

Side Effects of Endurance Training

It is not a race that we accomplish, but a journey we enjoy the most.

My journey has just begun, and there are miles to go before I sleep. With every breath during training, I release one negative thought out of my mind. The rebel in me has come out in full form, and I can feel the rush of energy. I am much more sorted and able to manage my mood swings better. I know how to unleash my stubborn thoughts. I have also evolved as a mother, and my children are a part of my workout regime. They keep a check on my runs and workout. As both my boys are into athletics, they can feel my aching muscles and then I am given special attention.

I suffer from Premenstrual dysphoric disorder (PMDD) is a health problem that is similar to premenstrual syndrome (PMS) but is more serious. PMDD causes severe irritability, depression, or anxiety in the week or two before your period starts. Proper diet, guided training and required medication had helped me tremendously in managing PMDD.

For You Mothers

Motherhood is a big responsibility, but more than taking care of others, it is imperative to first take care of yourself. We live in a patriarchal society, and a mother will always be questioned when it comes to her children's upbringing; ensure you draw a line there.

As a great follower of Bhagwat Gita, I always remember Arjun's state of mind whenever in a fix. On the battlefield, when he saw his near and dear ones, he was taken aback and started cursing himself. He doubted his abilities and intention. Krishna comes as his savior and tells him that he has to stand firm and fight for his kingdom. Loss or death should not bother him and is a part of his duty.

Similarly, to follow my dreams, I'll have to fight for my right. An outspoken and a rebel woman is not an acceptable figure in society. A mother who travels alone, leaves her children behind for her races, goes for cycle tours as an only woman, and participates in male-dominant sports, doesn't have a comfortable life. But it's the choices one makes and sticks to, that make all the difference.

PMDD hampers my training days and I am totally immobile during my periods. I have a bulky uterus, and I have to alter my speed while running to manage the sudden spike of pain in the abdomen. I am still not out of the dark phase and regularly see my therapist for healing sessions. Above all, I accept myself.

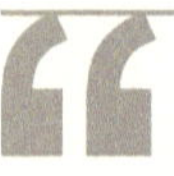*I must say, try the tri — it'll change you for good.*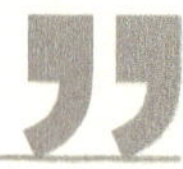

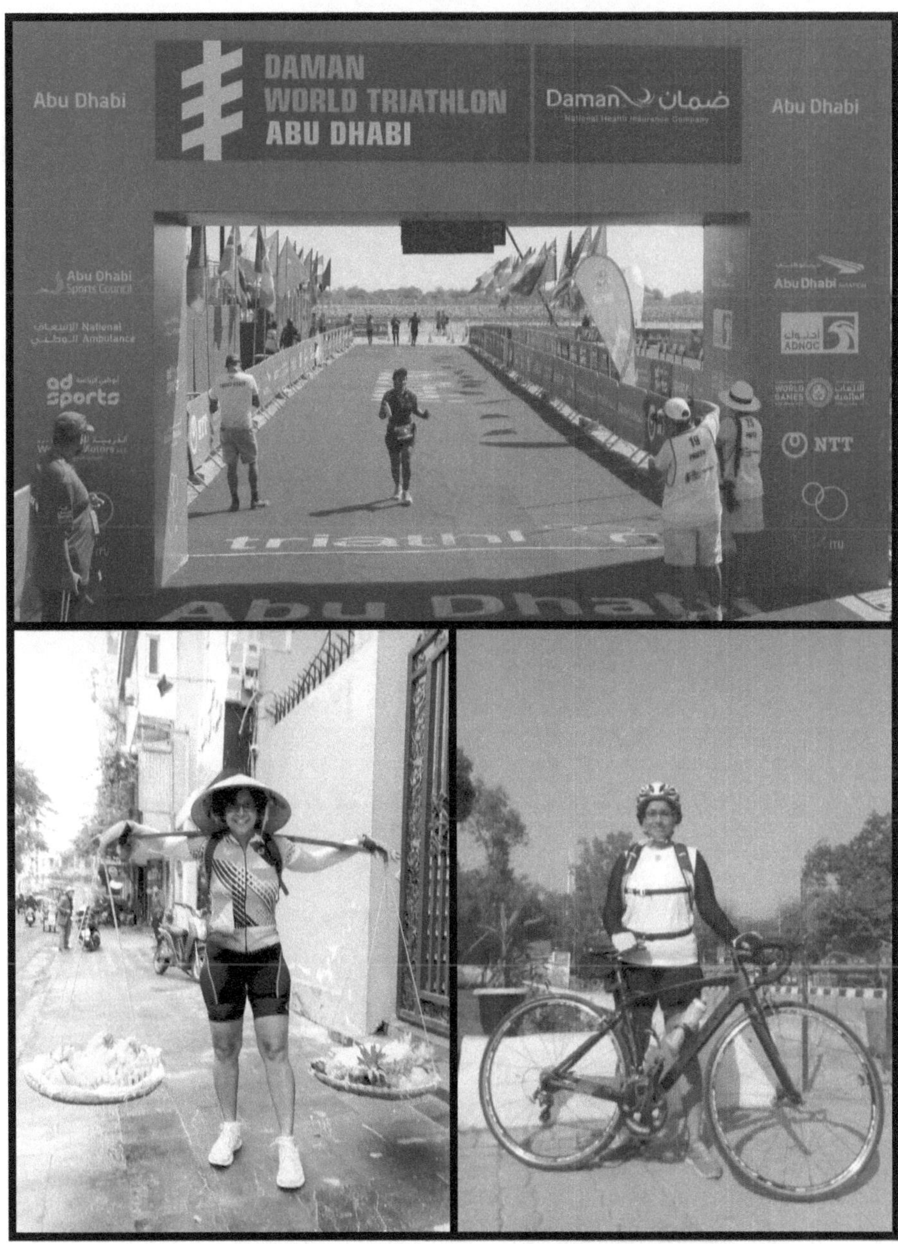
Abu Dhabi
DAMAN
WORLD TRIATHLON
ABU DHABI
Daman ضمان
National Health Insurance Company
Abu Dhabi
Abu Dhabi
Sports Council
National
Ambulance
ad
sports
Abu Dhabi
ADNOC
WORLD
GAMES
NTT
ITU
triathl

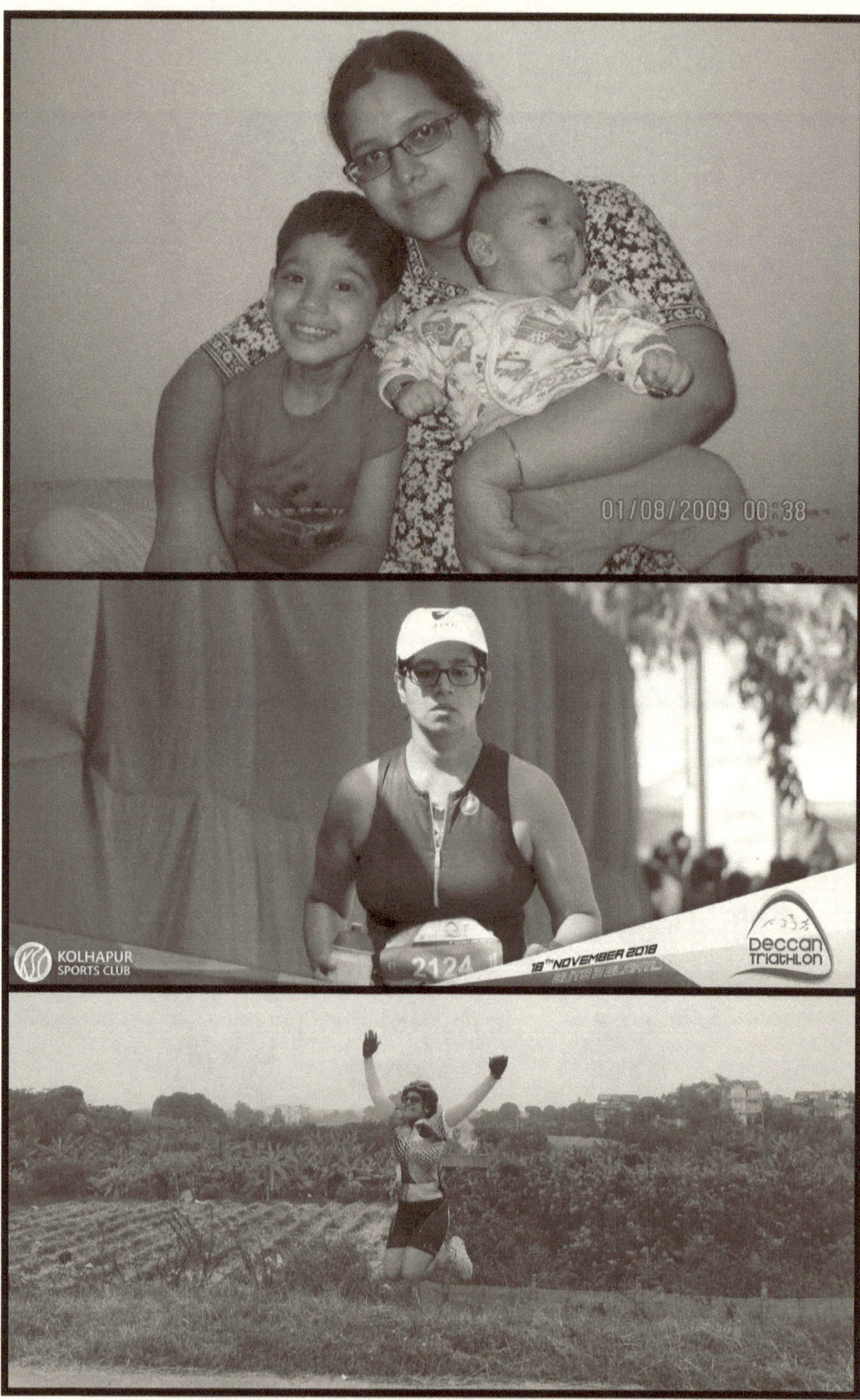

Quotes from the Coaches

Ritu has worked with me across multiple race formats, more recently the Full Marathon. But the most important race for her would be the Dubai IM70.3. Right from selecting a bike to working towards getting the swim on track. She put in hard efforts and it paid off in the end.

– Viv Menon, Mumbai
Coach – Ritu Kudal

Smithaa was already exceptional on the bike. We worked on her run and swim. Her consistency towards doing her workouts daily ensured her podiums in her category. It was a pleasure working with her.

– Viv Menon, Mumbai
Coach – Smithaa Kajale

To finish an Ironman is a great achievement in itself, it is even more inspiring when a 50+ year old woman does it. **Anjali**'s story is an inspiration to women of all ages that when you decide on giving yourself a challenge, with the right mindset you can make it happen.

– Kaustubh Radkar, Pune
Inspirational support for Anjali Bhalinge's Tri Journey

It takes a certain amount of mental toughness to complete an IM70.3 and dedication towards training for one. **Chandani** exhibited both and ensured she reached the finish line.

– Viv Menon, Mumbai
Coach – Chandani Desai

A tenacious, focused, no holds barred, true to herself, taskmaster, an endearing sports person, completely devoid of chicanery or subterfuge. A true student of pain and never say die attitude. Besides being a mother of two teenagers, a homemaker and a practicing Ophthalmologist. Kudos. Power to her…

– Dr. Harsh Shah, Sportsperson full time
(orthopedic surgeon in the spare time), Ahmedabad
(Uma's close friend who got her into the world of cycling)
Dr. Uma Vinod

I have been working with **Ami** for over three years now. Right from training her towards an HM. To subsequent Duathlons and Olympic Triathlons. She also loves her strength training sessions. More often than not she will get in touch with me and give me her week's schedule so that I can plan her workouts accordingly. Avid enthusiasts she is always ready to participate in BRMs, Duathlons and Triathlons. She is making steady progress and will definitely achieve her next goal. An IM 70.3.

– **Viv Menon, Mumbai**
Coach – Ami Paneri

What I love about coaching endurance athletes like **Charanya** is watching them change (mentally and physically) over the course of months from talking about the seemingly impossible to conquer their goals and inspiring others along the way."

– **Tim Wellman, Trilab Endurance, Texas**
Coach – Charanya

My Mommy Strongest

It's crazy how she can manage her job, me and my sister and training for the triathlons. It's inspiring to see something like her cause she's one in a million. I am proud to be her daughter. She is acheiving all her goals year after year, each one a little more difficult than the last. Her dedication is impeccable and her will to do something she has never ever thought of doing before is aspiring.

~ Soumya Kudal

Soumya & Diti,

(Ritu Kudal's daughters)

Pooja

(Anjali Bhalinge's daughter)

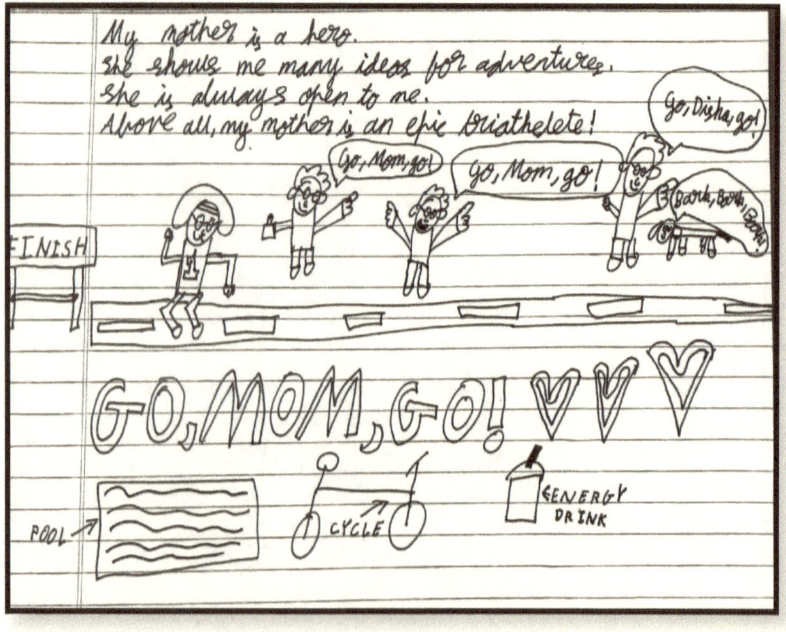

Shaurya

(Disha's younger son)

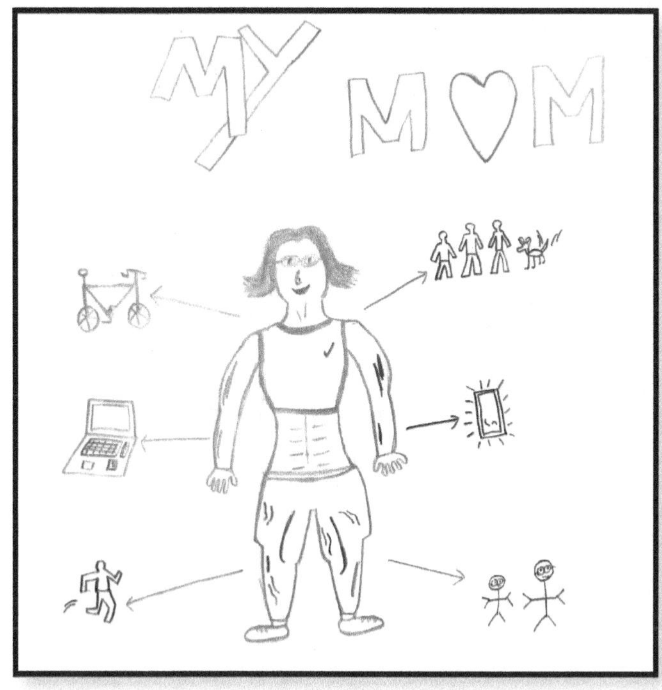

Siddhanth

(Disha's elder son)

My mom tri's because
I know she can-
My mom tri's because
she can do it.
My mom is dedicated
to her training
as a triathlete.
My mom is my role model
and my super hero!
Pranav
Son of Preeti.

About the Author

Disha, as her name suggests, is a multi-faceted lady.

A Mumbai based working mom, entrepreneur, enthusiastic athlete, passionate runner, an explorer on her bicycle, dance lover, insanely emotional, always high on life mother of two boys – Sid, Abhi and Tango (her pet dog).

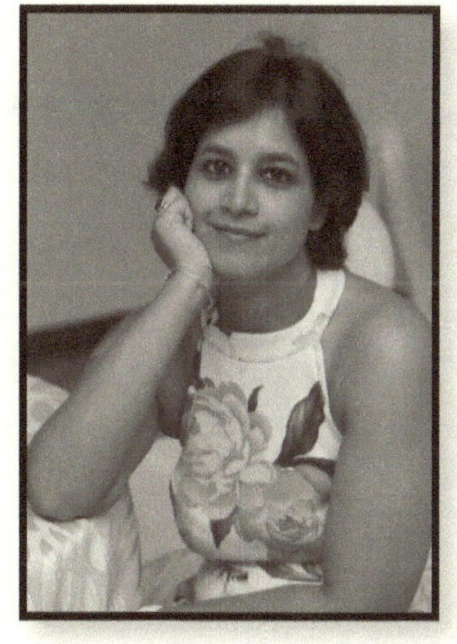

She believes in living life each day and finds magic in everything. Like, how the sky turns into shades of orange and varied colour at dusk and dawn, how butterflies flutter on flowers, how raindrops create a pattern on the puddle, how the wind blows her hair while cycling, how the sweat drips while running, how the muscles twitch while lifting weights.

She is a fighter in life and has taken the dark phase in her stride to evolve triumphantly.

She works in the development sector. Gender, Diversity & Inclusion and children are the causes close to her heart. She volunteers in several NGOs and story-telling to children is her favourite activity. She is a counsellor and a coach and practises voluntarily. She works closely with women, moreover mothers.

She loves to travel both solo and with her family. She is more of an experiential traveller and explores the world on her cycle. She runs a cycle tour company, "Atrangee" and encourages people to see and feel when they travel.

She has cycled far and wide on her bicycle, Amritsar to Wagah border, Bhutan, Rajasthan, Chattisgarh, Austria, Italy, Vietnam, to name a few.

She believes that anyone whom we meet has something to teach. She has a strong belief in womanhood's power, and she is an inspiration to many.

You can visit her site www.momthyname.blog and explore her world of freedom, happiness, enthusiasm, positivity and motivation.